T0223011

Routledge Revivals

Unwanted Pregnancy and Counselling

There was a growing concern in the 1970s about the number of unwanted pregnancies and the problems these posed for parents, children and society. Originally published in 1977, this was the first book which, with extensive reference to research material and illustrative case studies, provided a comprehensive analysis of the social and psychological background to unwanted pregnancy and a guide to ways of helping the people concerned. It should still be useful to doctors, nurses, midwives, teachers, social workers, and other professional and lay people whose work brings them into contact with those who are unhappy about a pregnancy.

Juliet Cheetham, whose previous contributions to the problem areas of social welfare are widely respected, discusses the different meanings of unwanted pregnancy, and goes on to explore its relationship to the changing position of women; to the role of the contemporary family; to the special problems experienced by natural children and their parents; to existing social and medical provisions. She examines the possibilities, risks and limitations of the various responses to unwanted pregnancy and the services available at the time, and analyses the difficulties men and women experience in using contraception.

Juliet Cheetham shows how the beliefs and attitudes of lay and professional people can influence their understanding of, and response to, these highly controversial and emotional subjects. She offers suggestions about the ways in which this influence may be appropriately modified, and the book concludes with a discussion of the special opportunities and problems of counselling those faced with an unwanted pregnancy.

Unwanted Pregnancy and Counselling

Juliet Cheetham

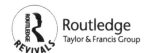

Routledge
Taylor & Francis Group

First published in 1977
by Routledge & Kegan Paul Ltd

This edition first published in 2022 by Routledge
2 Park Square, Milton Park, Abingdon, Oxon OX14 4RN

and by Routledge
605 Third Avenue, New York, NY 10158

Routledge is an imprint of the Taylor & Francis Group, an informa business

© 1977 Juliet Cheetham

Publisher's Note
The publisher has gone to great lengths to ensure the quality of this reprint but points out that some imperfections in the original copies may be apparent.

Disclaimer
The publisher has made every effort to trace copyright holders and welcomes correspondence from those they have been unable to contact.

A Library of Congress record exists under ISBN: 0710084994

ISBN: 978-1-032-11296-1 (hbk)
ISBN: 978-1-003-21931-6 (ebk)
ISBN: 978-1-032-11307-4 (pbk)

Book DOI 10.4324/9781003219316

Unwanted pregnancy and counselling

Juliet Cheetham

Routledge & Kegan Paul
London, Henley and Boston

First published in 1977
by Routledge & Kegan Paul Ltd
39 Store Street,
London WC1E 7DD,
Broadway House,
Newtown Road,
Henley-on-Thames,
Oxon RG9 1EN and
9 Park Street,
Boston, Mass. 02108, USA
Set in 10 on 12 point Times
and printed in Great Britain by
Lowe & Brydone Printers Ltd
Thetford, Norfolk

ISBN 0 7100 8499 4

To my parents and sister

Contents

five   Beliefs, attitudes and facts   86

six   Ways of helping   113

seven   **Aspects of counselling** 177

Bibliography

Index

Acknowledgments

It was originally intended that Eva Learner should be the co-author of this book. Although her numerous other commitments prevented this, she remained closely involved in planning its approach and contents. She also wrote some preliminary drafts. Her extensive experience of working with couples who are unhappy about a pregnancy, and her sympathy for them, helped me understand the complexity of their problems and put flesh on abstract theories. Her enthusiasm for the subject sustained me throughout the book's preparation.

My interest in unwanted pregnancy was greatly stimulated by my colleagues on the Lane Committee; I learnt much from their disciplined approach to their work. I also owe a special debt of gratitude to the many men and women who were good enough to talk to me about their own experiences of unwanted pregnancy.

My discussions with Pauline Crabbe and David Paintin deepened my knowledge of counselling those faced with this problem. I have tried to convey something of their understanding and skills in the last chapter.

Margaret Adcock, Jane Aldgate, Ellis Christopher, Alan Fox, Betty Hill, Michael Hill and Alec Turnbull read parts of the manuscript and I am grateful for their criticisms and encouragement. I wish this book could adequately reflect their expertise in their particular fields. I would also like to thank Margaret Bramall, Ann Cartwright, Michael Fogden, François Lafitte, Doreen Rothman and the staff of the British Pregnancy Advisory Service for their efficient response to requests for information.

Gillian Bowles, with skill, speed and good humour, transformed numerous indecipherable drafts into the final manuscript.

As always, it was my family who helped me most: my mother and sister by looking after my children on many occasions; my children by their generous understanding of my preoccupation; my husband by taking the lion's share of our domestic responsibilities and still finding time to correct the manuscript. The book could never have been completed without him and I shamefully exploited his patience and good will.

Juliet Cheetham

one

Introduction and basic assumptions

Extreme nervousness dominated her, a kind of suppressed hysteria; her cheeks were flushed and her eyes red-rimmed; she had been weeping. . . .

On a sudden she clutched his arm . . . fixing him with a terrified stare: 'Ah knew it'd happen. . . . Ah knew it'd happen.'. . .

'We should ne'er ha' done it. . . . Ah've bin feard for a fortnight. . . . Ah went t' t' doctor at dinner time. . . . He told me. . . . Ah'm, – y'know.'

His mouth opened; he swallowed hard, and blinked.

Fearfully she gripped his arm tighter and said, in low, scared, tones: 'What shall we do, Harry . . .?'

He felt choked, staring back at her, a freezing sensation creeping up his body. He could find no words (*Love on the Dole*, W. Greenwood, 1975, p. 179).

She was distinctly conscious now of the birth of a new feeling of love for the coming child – the child which to some extent existed for her already – and she abandoned herself to it blissfully. The child was no longer only a part of her body but sometimes lived his own independent life. Often this was the cause of suffering but at the same time her strange new joy made her want to laugh aloud (*Anna Karenin*, L.N. Tolstoy, 1973, p. 702).

My soul doth magnify the Lord (Luke 1 : 46).

Women may long for pregnancy or they may dread it. It may be a time of supreme happiness and expectation or of fear and loneliness. That there have always been many pregnancies and children that are not only unplanned or untimely but are, and continue to be, unwanted is clear from the high rates of infanticide and gross neglect of children which were, until this century, a part of daily experience, and which still have not disappeared. But only during the last fifty years or so has unwanted pregnancy become a matter of open public concern.

The origins of this new consciousness are complex. In part it reflects a growing desire and ability to control aspects of human life and suffering which had formerly to be accepted with resignation. Happiness, or having what you want, are now commonly seen to be rights, rather than distant ideals or the ultimate rewards of effort and achievement. From these aspirations and increasing human ingenuity have come the solution of some problems and the creation of others. Nowhere is this more clearly illustrated than in the field of human reproduction.

Huge drops in infant mortality and greatly increased life expectancy, as well as advances in medicine and social welfare, have brought with them a population explosion which is far from being controlled by developments in contraception. In its turn, the possibility of controlling fertility, although usually accepted as an unqualified blessing, brings its own problems. It challenges women to contemplate social roles other than full-time motherhood. Acceptance of this challenge threatens prevailing assumptions about family life and about equality. Efforts to maintain the status quo frustrate women's aspirations and achievements. Discontent and conflict may be necessary preliminaries to human advancement but they are not comfortable to live with.

With decreasing family size has come a lively awareness of children's emotional and material needs which can in part be met by greater public and private wealth. And yet children are still unloved and neglected and parents tormented by their failure to provide adequate homes and care. Some of these children are both unplanned and unwanted. This condition, although as old as life itself, now seems more intolerable because, with efficient methods of contraception, it could be prevented; but contraception is not always effective and often is not used.

The last resort for those who cannot contemplate responsibility for unwanted children is, and always has been, abortion, which in Britain, until less than a decade ago, was nearly always illegal. Many, perhaps most, unwanted pregnancies are not terminated, but the legalisation of abortion, in its deliberate weighing of the quality of life against the destruction of life or the potential for life, brings complex questions to the fore. What is an unwanted pregnancy? Who does not want it, and when, and why? What is the relationship between unwanted pregnancy and unwanted children? What happens to unwanted children?

Defining unwanted pregnancy

Except for the purposes of research, exact definitions are less important than clarity about the different meanings which can be attached to the adjective 'unwanted'. Although there are pregnancies which are so clearly and unambiguously wanted that they prompt no doubts, no hesitation about their outcome and no mixed feelings, it is usually mistaken to equate wanting, or not wanting, with unqualified pleasure or dismay. More commonly, pregnancy is accompanied by varying degrees of enthusiasm and apprehension, feelings which change with the different stages of the pregnancy and with visions of the immediate or more distant future (Pohlman, 1965). A woman may want to be a mother, or parents may want another child, while at the same time realising that their circumstances would make it impossible for them to provide the quality of life they believe to be necessary. Although it may seem a remote abstraction to talk of 'society' not wanting a child, such a conclusion can be drawn when political, economic and social conditions appear to be inimical to people's desire for children.

'Unwanted pregnancy' can therefore have many different and valid meanings. This is a complicated and muddled world where unplanned pregnancies may be wanted, where wanted children may emerge from unwanted pregnancies, where the offspring of wanted pregnancies may be rejected, where infatuation with infants grows cold and where children may be wanted solely to meet their parents' pathological needs. These problems are compounded by the fact that although there are numerous hypotheses about the implications of unwanted pregnancy for parents and children, these cannot usually be confirmed or denied by reliable research evidence (Pohlman, 1969).

Whatever might be the achievements of social policy, education and medical practice, it is impossible to imagine a world in which all pregnancies were unequivocally welcomed by the couples concerned. This book is concerned not only with the minority whose difficulties are so acute that the pregnancy is terminated, or the mother parts with her child, but also with the needs of those couples for whom pregnancy means considerable ambivalence, perhaps because of the reordering of their lives and values a child will entail. These conflicts are a part of human experience, and for some, an essential step in their progress towards maturity. The fact that they are so commonplace does not mean that the people concerned should be left to resolve them alone. Indecision, resentment, anxiety, self-doubt and recrimination are painful and debilitating, and their effects can be widespread.

Some basic assumptions

An underlying theme of much of the discussion in this book is the relationship between social, economic and political conditions, and individuals' aspirations and achievements. There is no presumption either that the material world inevitably and always moulds an individual's destiny and personality or that people can remain unaffected by their environment. Each influences the other in subtle and complex ways.

From this assumption it is argued that unwanted pregnancy and reactions to it can only be properly understood in the context of changing male and female roles, of the functions of the family, and of current beliefs about state and individual responsibility. Because these are highly contentious subjects it follows that there will be no exact fit between what appears to be the professed will of the majority and policies giving concrete expression to this will. It would, for example, now be unusual to hear explicit statements that single parents or natural children should be treated less well than other families; indeed, it is frequently affirmed that their vulnerability entitles them to privileged treatment. Nevertheless, despite this apparent good will, they remain among the poorest members of the community. This is partly because the policies necessary to improve their situation appear, in the short term at least, to be expensive; minorities are not usually powerful enough to force the majority to put its ideals into practice when this entails some redistribution of resources from the better to the less well off. These policies also fail to attract widespread support because they challenge prevailing assumptions about marriage and family life.

Similarly, the wide-ranging policies necessary to reduce the number of unwanted pregnancies, policies involving education, housing and welfare, medical practice and positive discrimination for working women, seem too high a price to pay. People prefer what appear to be simple, more short-term solutions, for example, adoption, or abortion, or the more efficient use of contraception. All these things can contribute to solving the problems of unwanted pregnancy, but as later chapters will show, to the individuals concerned they are rarely simple solutions. And unwanted pregnancy is still far from being an uncommon problem. Two questions therefore need always to be asked about policies which purport to reduce the incidence of unwanted pregnancy: do they take proper account of the complexity of this problem and are they likely to attract practical support rather than vague and insubstantial goodwill?

Implicit in these questions is the conscious weighing of the possibility, within existing structures, of happiness and an adequate standard of living for a child and his parents. When this possibility is remote abortion is now accepted by many as the lesser evil. The author shares this view and sees abortion as providing one legitimate, although often only partial, solution to the problems which surround unwanted pregnancy.

At times this book may seem to perpetuate the long tradition of discussing pregnancy, childbirth and the care of infants as if these were exclusively the concerns of women. This tradition is a bad one. There is considerable evidence that, despite all kinds of discouragement, men feel greatly involved in these matters. This increasing involvement will be both the cause and result of continuing changes in the aspirations and roles of both sexes, and therefore in their respective rights and responsibilities as parents. If this book does not seem to give sufficient weight to this, the reason is because its chief concern is with the ends and means of helping individuals with the immediate problems which surround unwanted pregnancy. And it is still true that women bear most, if not all, the responsibility of deciding what to do about an unwanted pregnancy; and for many the responsibilities of parenthood are theirs alone (Finer Report, 1974, vol. 1). This fact, as well as the experience of pregnancy and childbirth, means that male and female perspectives of a mother's situation will often differ, and account should be taken of this. Proclaiming the equality of the sexes must not include denying differences; it means, among other things, giving special attention and help to those who carry the greatest burdens.

It may be argued that too much attention is being devoted to the problems rather than to the pleasures of pregnancy and child care. Do not most women, on balance, welcome their pregnancies? Is there not a danger of inventing or exaggerating difficulties? Although the answer to the first question is probably yes, in Britain, as elsewhere in the world, very large numbers of unwanted pregnancies still occur every year. In answer to the second question, subsequent chapters will show that the problems that surround these pregnancies are often real and acute but more likely to be ignored than exaggerated. People who are denied understanding, attention, compassion, and, above all, practical help are unlikely to feel very positive about themselves or their dependants. This means a sad legacy for the next generation.

The incidence of unwanted pregnancy

How common is it for pregnancy to be in some degree and at some stage unwanted? Caplan (1957, p. 26) reports that 80 per cent of women he studied who were expecting their first baby 'admitted conscious feelings of marked disappointment and anxiety when they found they had become pregnant'. He argues elsewhere (1961) that the extent to which their pregnancies will be an experience of personal growth and their children welcome depends on how these disappointments and anxieties are handled.

Cartwright (1970) found that, amongst the mothers she studied, a fifth had had one pregnancy which at the time they did not want at all, and another quarter had a pregnancy earlier than they wanted. Bone's (1973) study revealed that probably over a third of each year's pregnancies to married women or women living in a stable cohabitation were unplanned, and about half of these were unwanted in the sense that the mothers 'were sorry it had happened at all'. In a later study Cartwright (1976) found that the proportion of mothers who regretted their pregnancies in these terms rose from one in twenty of those having their first or second child to a third of those having their third and just over half having their fourth or later child.

In 1961 over 65,000 natural children were born. It would be quite wrong to assume that all these children were the result of unwanted pregnancies. Many of the parents concerned live in stable cohabitations with the same chances of planning pregnancies as married couples. Moreover, some single women wish to become pregnant, or decide they would like to have a baby even though they have not planned the pregnancy (Macintyre, 1976b). Nevertheless, a substantial proportion of natural children are both unplanned and unwanted. This is especially likely when their mothers are young, and today very many children are born to single women less than twenty years old.

In 1973 over 110,000 pregnancies of women resident in Britain were terminated. A tiny minority of these will have been planned and terminated because a serious foetal abnormality has been detected, but the vast majority are unplanned and, for a variety of reasons, unwanted.

Although it would be impossible to calculate the total number of unwanted pregnancies the figures we have show that every year many thousands of men and women face the anxiety and anguish this entails, and that many thousands of children are born into a situation where they will be at best vulnerable, and at worst severely handicapped. What might be done to reduce this suffering?

A partial answer to this question can be found in the various welfare and medical provisions discussed in chapter 6. It is also argued that these services will often not be appropriately used unless the individuals concerned receive some counselling.

All this help is crucially important and often neglected. But in many important senses it is designed to cope with, rather than to prevent, the casualties of a social system which, as chapters 2 and 4 argue, is bound to produce large numbers of unwanted pregnancies. While we may have some understanding of the mechanisms of this system, it is much more difficult to imagine how, in practical terms, it might be made to function less destructively. Some of the changes required could mean a radical transformation of society, a transformation which will probably bring a new set of problems. It is sometimes said, for example, that not only do women as workers need to be given equal opportunities with men, but that the status and rewards, including the economic rewards, of motherhood must be vastly increased if society is not to endorse, explicitly and implicitly, the view that it is primarily in employment outside the home that the greatest prestige is to be found. Such supports for motherhood, if they were more than nominal, might reduce the number of unwanted pregnancies. They would also require a society oriented far more towards reproduction than production, a difficult state to achieve in a world dominated by rising material aspirations, and one which might also mean a greatly increased birthrate.

Any honest exploration of the background to unwanted pregnancy and of the solutions proposed must reveal inconsistencies and injustices inherent in our social arrangements. Before these can be tackled they must be questioned and this questioning may well prompt an individual to choose a course of action which does not fit easily with conventional expectations. Adjustment to these standards is not necessarily helpful. Only by challenging and redefining needs and expectations can new equilibriums be achieved. 'It remains true that one major limit to the possibility of change is the capacity to envisage it' (Oakley, 1974b, p. 197).

The ends and means of counselling

These new perspectives may have their origins in counselling but what are usually seen to be its more immediate purposes? Briefly, counselling in relation to unwanted pregnancy involves providing the woman or couple with opportunities to discuss their problems, as they see them, with someone they trust; to explore the background to these difficulties, and to consider the possible alternatives before them so that, bearing in mind the inevitable conflicting interests, they may choose the one with which they can be most at peace. It also means helping people marshal the resources available in such a way that they can pursue as effectively as possible the course of action they have chosen.

Counselling is based on the assumption that there is value in the free expression of both painful and pleasurable feelings and in the honest examination of conflicts; and that there is a relationship between these processes and future behaviour less damaging to individuals and those concerned with them. Although most counsellors will probably agree with these general statements, depending on their definitions of problems and their moral view-point, their practical interpretation varies considerably.

Given the very large numbers of people facing unwanted pregnancies and their differing needs it is highly desirable that counsellors from many different backgrounds should be involved with them. Doctors, nurses, health visitors, social workers, teachers, youth workers, clergy and lay counsellors are likely to be concerned with this problem at some stage in their careers. All their different interpretations of counselling will have something to offer some individuals, but this book is intended to help counsellors to think more clearly about the relationship between their own objectives and methods and the actual problems surrounding the unwanted pregnancy of the particular individuals they are trying to help. This flexibility is important not only because of differing needs but because there is as yet little research evidence to demonstrate which counselling method is most effective in which situations (Illsley and Hall, 1974, p. 19).

The case for counselling

The advent of legal abortion has prompted considerable discussion about the need for counselling those faced with an unwanted pregnancy. This was strongly endorsed by the Lane Committee on the working of the Abortion Act and the Select Committee set up to examine amendments to the abortion law. There is also widespread support for counselling from many professional organisations. Despite all this the counselling help available is often inadequate.

It is difficult to assess the shortcomings accurately because so many different people, can at various stages, be concerned with a woman who is unhappy about her pregnancy. Existing studies mostly concern women asking for abortions who are only a minority of those who could be helped by counselling (Cartwright and Lucas, 1974; Ingham and Simms, 1972; Williams and Hindell, 1972). Nevertheless, these studies show that a large number of women feel they have few opportunities for helpful discussion about their problems and that it can be particularly difficult for them to talk to hospital doctors. When their consultations have been brusque and unsympathetic, or merely brisk and superficial, many women feel that an event of great importance to them has been trivialised. Studies discussed in chapters 4 and 6 also show that it is common for unmarried mothers to feel that they receive only grudging help and inadequate information, and that often at the price of admonishment for supposed sexual misdemeanours. Several organisations such as the National Child Birth Trust argue, as Kitzinger (1962) and Caplan (1961) have done, that there is inadequate support and counselling for most pregnant women, whatever their circumstances, and that this can mean, at worst, greater problems during and after pregnancy and, at best, missed opportunities for emotional development.

The evidence given by numerous organisations to the Lane

Committee and the research carried out on behalf of that Committee reveal that many professionals are also concerned about the inadequacies of their counselling help, inadequacies they see as being connected with lack of both time and skill. Although describing the work of doctors, Main's lucid account of their problems could be extended to all counsellors confronted by women worried about their pregnancies.

> These had led the doctors variously to indignant refusal, argument, parental type admonition, warnings, hasty routine signings of the form (giving consent for termination of pregnancy), placatory agreement, indulgent protectiveness and other emotional responses but rarely to cool surveys ... [of the problem] (1971, p. 55).

Why is it so common for only lip service to be paid to the value of counselling? The first obstacle seems to be the belief that counselling inevitably forms an integral part of all professionals' work. Counselling in this sense often means little more than treating people with courtesy and respect which, in spite of much evidence to the contrary, all professionals think they do anyway. Given these assumptions, further efforts to provide counselling are unnecessary.

The second obstacle is the view that although counselling may provide comfort for some women, and therefore a more humane service, it is a largely unnecessary luxury to be dispensed with when time and resources are scarce. What is needed is proper medical and welfare services and counselling is not thought to be an integral part of these.

A less obvious but no less potent obstacle is the fear that counselling, which means getting close to individuals and seeing their problems and their strengths and weaknesses in all their complexity, will make it harder to be content with simple, inflexible solutions. Professional helpers will then have to bear the burden of recognising that the help they or anyone else can offer may well be inadequate. They will also be challenged to abandon comforting stereotypes of women who are anxious about their pregnancies as unfeeling monsters, whose sole wish is to dispose of their children, or as poor unfortunates, victims only of social circumstances and predatory males.

What, then, is the case for counselling? First and foremost

counselling is an essential part of the process of understanding the problems surrounding an unwanted pregnancy and, therefore, of arriving at the most appropriate course of action. Common sense alone tells us that failure to hear what people are saying, or trying to say, about their circumstances will lead to mistaken diagnosis and unnecessary or harmful treatment. The Lane Committee heard from many women who felt their predicament had been entirely ignored or who had been rushed into making inappropriate decisions. This is confirmed by Horobin *et al.* (1973) who found that some doctors tended to believe that unwanted pregnancy was more easily managed by poor working-class women than by women higher up the social scale. This conclusion was based on dubious sociological generalisations about the acceptability of illegitimacy, which meant that they failed to ask for, or to listen carefully to, working-class women's accounts of their circumstances. When these women and their problems were examined by independent assessors it was found that their doctors' prejudices had left some of the most disturbed women from the poorest backgrounds coping with pregnancies and the care of their offspring in extremely unpromising circumstances. By contrast, more capable middle-class women, with more resources, had been given abortions. Horobin *et al.* also thought that the relative contentment of both those whose request for abortion had been refused as well as those whose request had been granted was associated with the fact that they felt their difficulties had been fully and sympathetically considered.

Counselling at the point of crisis also seems to make it more likely that people will return more readily for other help they may need. The clearest evidence of this comes from studies of women who have had abortions and who felt they were given adequate counselling. Women who have been sympathetically treated and who understand the nature of the operation and its implications are more likely to return for post-operative check-ups and con- traceptive help. Counselling has also been found to play a significant role in helping women undergo out-patient abortion which minimises the need for anaesthesia (Lewis *et al.*, 1971).

For those who believe that the morality of certain acts depends partly on how far the implications of these have been fully considered counselling may have some moral significance. This aspect of counselling and its problems and opportunites are now widely recognised (Halmos, 1969; North, 1972). It must, of course, be distinguished from attempts to influence someone towards a particular moral view point against his or her better judgment, and without examination of possible alternatives.

Last, but by no means least, several studies have shown that women want and value counselling help. although naturally enough there are many different views about what should be its ends and means. Rather than being an invasion of women's rights it is a means of identifying and disentangling the numerous choices confronting a woman with an unwanted pregnancy (Ingham and Simms, 1972; Horobin *et al.*, 1973; Cartwright and Lucas, 1974; Illsley and Hall, 1974).

The contents of this book

The interest and relevance of this book's different sections will vary according to the knowledge and expertise of particular groups of counsellors. The following brief accounts of the contents is therefore intended to help readers to be selective.

Chapter 2 examines, primarily from a sociological perspective, the relationship between unwanted pregnancy and the changing roles of men and women and the functions of the family. This may appear an unusual analysis for counsellors more used to defining problems and their solutions in entirely individual terms; but the main argument of the chapter is that such definitions will be inadequate if they are divorced from a broad social context.

The third chapter discusses psychological aspects of pregnancy and motherhood, about which there are many theories but few facts. The possible relationships between the outer and inner worlds of individuals are explored, with pregnancy and early motherhood being seen as potentially providing opportunities for emotional growth, and for resolving earlier difficulties.

Chapter 4 examines the circumstances of parents and children who face special difficulties, for example single or very young mothers. The complex origins of these difficulties and their implications are also discussed.

Chapter 5 looks at the ways in which beliefs and attitudes about the highly contentious issues associated with unwanted pregnancy influence medical and welfare services, as well as the work of counsellors. This chapter may be of particular importance to those who think the help they give is scrupulously objective.

The sixth chapter describes various kinds of help available to couples facing an unwanted pregnancy. These descriptions only provide basic guidelines, together with the information about sources of more specialist knowledge for counsellors unfamiliar with these services.

The last chapter discusses in some detail the ends, means and particular problems of counselling those people who are anxious or unhappy about a pregnancy.

two

Women, pregnancy and motherhood in their social context

Longer life, sex ratio near unity, more and younger marriages and small consciously planned families, with fertility compressed into a narrow band of years, have resulted in revolutionary alterations in women's lives as wives, as mothers and as workers (Finer Report, 1974, Vol 1, para. 3. 18).

Total liberation from the constraints of a divisively feminine upbringing in a decidedly sexist culture implies such an unrealistically optimistic view of the human capacity to change that it is probably never possible (Oakley, 1974b, p. 195).

It is within the context of these dramatic changes in women's roles and the inevitable conflicts these mean, for both men and women, that attitudes towards sex, pregnancy and child bearing must be understood.

In tracing these relationships and their implications for individual men and women this chapter draws extensively from the literature on women's position in society, a literature which is rapidly expanding with renewed interest in feminism.

Women as wives and mothers

Motherhood used to be a woman's whole existence; it has become now the lesser part of the chronology of her life cycle (Finer Report, 1974, Vol. 1, para. 3. 19).

During the last sixty years marriage has become increasingly popular and the average age of men and women when they marry decreases almost annually. Only a quarter of women aged twenty to twenty-four were married in 1901 but more than half of them in 1966. Family size has also decreased and the life expectation of men and women has risen dramatically. The details of these changes can be found in Halsey (1972a) and the Finer Report but, briefly, the implications for men and women are that they can expect to spend more than fifty years of their lives married with only half or less of this period devoted to the care and upbringing of children. Since children tend to be born during the first few years of marriage, for only six or seven years will a married woman have pre-school children to care for. Compared with a typical working-class mother in the 1890s, who would spend about fifteen years either pregnant or nursing a baby, the average woman today will spend only four years in this state, and her family is likely to be completed during the first ten years of her marriage before she is thirty (Titmuss, 1963, pp. 91–2).

How have women and society reacted to this 'gift of time' (Myrdal and Klein, 1968) which would have seemed so extraordinary to their grandparents? Answers to this question must take account of two important and, at times, apparently conflicting trends. The first is the preoccupation with children's many needs, and the responsibilities of their parents, and particularly of their mothers, to meet these; the second is the growing awareness of many of these mothers, no matter now devoted they are to their children, of the emotional and social costs of child rearing in an industrial society.

Radical improvements in children's health and material welfare have been accompanied by increasingly sophisticated views about their intellectual and emotional needs. Paradoxically, the provisions of a welfare state enlarge rather than diminish parents' responsibilities. The implications are that

> Society is in the process of making parenthood a highly self conscious, self regarding affair. In doing so it is adding to the sense of responsibility among parents. Their tasks are much harder and involve more risks of failure when children have to be brought up as individual successes .... Bringing up children becomes less a matter of rule of thumb, custom and tradition; more a matter of acquired knowledge and expert advice. More decisions have to be made because there is so much more to be decided; and as the margin of felt responsibility extends so does the scope for anxiety about one's children (Titmuss, 1963, p. 9).

Titmuss describes these responsibilities as shared between parents. Many studies, including those of the Newsons (1965 and 1970), have shown that partly because of decreasing hours of work, and partly because of changes in views about the roles of men and women, fathers now take a greater part in the upbringing of their children. Nevertheless, during children's pre-school years it is mothers who carry the primary responsibility for their care (Oakley, 1974b). To them fall the satisfactions and frustrations and the hard work that this involves; and since many families now live away from their relatives, who previously would have shared in the care of small children, women may have to carry these responsibilities without much or any support.

This relatively new pattern of family life produces and is sustained by beliefs that mothers and children have an almost exclusive need for each other and that motherhood is a woman's greatest and most rewarding achievement. Although they do not find it easy to be frank about their doubts, women are becoming much less sure about these assertions as they come to see motherhood as only one of their many possible roles, as one phase in their lives (Oakley, 1974b; Gavron, 1968; J. and E. Newson, 1965 and 1970).

The first phase is devoted to education and to full-time employment or higher education before marriage. After marriage many women may continue to work full time for a few years but then move into the second phase – that of motherhood. For most women this is a full-time occupation, at least until their last child goes to school, and it marks a radical change in the quality and style of her life. For the first time, since she herself was a small child, her world will be bounded by the walls of her own home and she will be economically completely dependent on her husband. Many women welcome this change and are glad to devote themselves for a few years to the care of small children. Others, perhaps an increasing number, are surprised to find that this period which they had been encouraged to see as the supreme moment in their lives is at times tedious and frustrating. Often they feel ill-prepared for the difficult tasks of child-rearing. Those women who move into the third phase – that of retirement from full-time 'active motherhood' – and return to work have about twenty-five to thirty working years before them.

With foresight, careful planning, the support of relatives and an adequate income, potentially this is a life of considerable variety and many different satisfactions. It also has inherent risks. Women who have been encouraged to pursue a sophisticated education in the expectation that they will follow responsible careers may, when they have children, find it increasingly difficult to continue this objective for a variety of reasons, including prejudice against the employment of married women, especially mothers. All kinds of constraints, in the employment of women, in the provision of substitute care for children and in social attitudes, may make choice illusory rather than real. Other women may feel conflicts of loyalty when they see that their husbands and children want the major share of their energy and attention while they long for some of the financial and emotional independence of work. Doubts about what is entailed in giving children the best possible physical and emotional care prompts anxieties about the implications of a mother's employment outside the home. Visions of alternative roles and a high standard of living combined with the expectation that fertility can be controlled make it likely that unplanned pregnancies will increasingly be seen as unwanted, not to be accepted with resignation.

These difficulties encourage women to think ahead no further than the immediate future and to abandon themselves to the role which is fully accepted, though not fully supported, by society, that of preoccupied motherhood. For many families there are definite advantages in the commitment, provided it is accepted that it will usually only be satisfying for the woman, and accepted by her children, for a relatively short period of her life. The costs of fostering intensive contacts no longer wanted or needed by a mother or her child are frightening.

It should be more widely recognised that it is in the very nature of a mother's position in our society to avenge her own frustrations on a small, helpless child; whether this takes the form of tyranny or of smothering affection that asks the child to be a substitute for all she has missed (Fraser, 1968, p. 153).

Women as workers

None but a fool will take a wife whose bread must be earned solely by his labour and who will contribute nothing towards it herself (*Present for a Serving Maid 1743*, George, 1925, p. 168).

Women have to live two lives and they must learn to play
the different and often conflicting roles of mothers and workers.
They are taught the lesson, too, that formal equality is
mocked by the practical inequalities of the labour market
where women still serve as the main reserve of cheap labour
(Finer Report, 1974, para. 3. 23).

Well over a third of Britain's work force is female. Nearly a half
of all married women are in paid employment as are 40 per cent
of those with dependent children, including nearly a fifth of those
mothers with children aged four or less. These proportions have
all increased dramatically within the last twenty-five years (Hunt,
1968; DEP, 1974, 1975).

Pressures for women to work come from two main sources: the
needs of several industries and professions and the wish of many
women to be in paid employment. In spite of economic recessions
there has been a continuous demand for women workers, not least
because of their preparedness to take on the lowest paid jobs, for
example, in the retail and catering industries, and for female
clerks and secretaries. The well-being of many people also
depends on the large numbers of women employed in the 'caring
professions' of nursing, teaching and social work. With work no
longer being seen as merely a prelude to marriage women become
skilled and experienced members of the labour force.

Married women's desire for work arises partly from economic
necessity. Increases in the cost of living accompanied by rising
expectations of acceptable standards make it imperative for some
women and desirable for others to contribute to the family income. It is also associated with a perception of paid employment,
however menial, as providing status, companionship and
fulfilment not to be found in domesticity (Jephcott et al., 1962;
Klein, 1965). These rewards are even greater for the steadily
increasing number of women with professional and technical
qualifications, and they seem to outweigh the personal and practical hardships of working and rearing a family simultaneously.

Attitudes towards the employment of women endorse these
trends. It is now accepted that although mothers with young
children need to be protected from pressures to work and may
require special consideration if they are to be employed, it is
neither right nor possible to exempt all women, on the strength of
their potential or completed motherhood, from the general ex-

pectation of society that its able-bodied members will be economically productive. To do so in an industrial society, with its rift between home and workplace, its mass production of such goods as food and clothing and its centralised education and welfare services, would deprive women of opportunities to be productive members of society, except in so far as they are fully employed in the rearing of young children. There is little honour or fulfilment in being a parasite (Myrdal and Klein, 1968).

Those who are critical of many of the features of capitalist society may regret the willingness of women to sell their labour, often in conditions of exploitation. Nevertheless, the fact that so many are eager to do this is a reflection of the comparatively greater dissatisfactions women seem to experience if they are confined entirely to domestic routine with its long hours of physically tiring and frequently tedious work for no material reward. In spite of the emotional satisfactions a woman may find in this labour, especially if it is openly appreciated by her family, it is extremely hard for most people to feel properly valued members of society without some financial recognition of their services. While society extols the virtues of motherhood, the tangible rewards it offers mothers are few. They are expected to find their satisfactions privately.

How far is experience of work after they have had children anticipated by women and what priority does it assume for them? There are only a few studies relevant to this question, and since attitudes are changing quickly, these findings need to be supplemented by personal observations.

Klein (1965) found that the lives of the women in her study were dominated by their actual or expected role as wives and mothers. Their homes and their families were the focal point of their interests and these were regarded by themselves and by others as their main responsibility. All other responsibilities were subordinate to this central function. There appeared to be no feeling that women ought to work or had the right to do this; they did so largely of their own volition to use up surplus energy. The return of women to work did not appear to be premeditated and it occurred in circumstances which seem to have been unforeseen, although not unforeseeable. Klein argues that this approach to work does not accord with the facts of women's employment.

These attitudes may be less typical of highly educated women, especially those who have completed their education, many of whom expect only a brief interruption in their careers when they have children, and who may postpone having children until they are sufficiently established in their careers to make this feasible. These women do not reject domestic and family life. On the contrary, they value family life highly; their marriages are generally happy and they are conscientious mothers who will only accept the highest quality substitute care for their children. While willing to delegate many household chores they are anxious to retain as much responsibility as possible for the more personal aspects of family life such as cooking and child care. These dual-career couples, although a tiny minority, deserve attention as pioneers in working out new relationships between work and family responsibilities (Collins, 1964; Arreggar, 1966; Fogarty *et al.*, 1971; R. and R. N. Rapoport, 1971).

For many women the satisfactions of the worlds of work and home are best achieved by working part time. As a consequence it is common to find that although men's career aspirations rise with time and the transition into family responsibilities, for women this trend is reversed (Williams, 1969).

Women's attitudes to work have also been coloured by the fact that they have been regarded to a large extent as a reserve labour force who, because they are so frequently supported by their husbands, do not need the same conditions of work as men. With relatively insecure and unrewarding work they tend therefore to live a somewhat vicarious life with their status, prestige and satisfaction dependent on the achievements of their husbands and children rather than on the quality or quantity of their own paid work.

The Equal Pay and Sex Discrimination Acts are intended to remedy some of these iniquities but in so far as they promise more than can immediately be achieved they may increase the frustrations of many women. They certainly endorse the value of women as workers rather than as mothers.

Women and education

> When we were growing up many of us could not see
> ourselves beyond the age of twenty-one. We had no image of
> our own future, of ourselves as women (Friedan, 1971, p. 69).

An individual's education cannot be understood only in terms of experience in schools and colleges because these are indelibly influenced by the person's self-image, by his or her expectations of the future. Parental or family interpretations of various, often conflicting, social pressures to some extent shape these expectations. They act as a filter, leaving the child more or less exposed to the chance of conforming with conventional expectations of his or her role, or of redefining these according to individual taste. What are these pressures?

Attitudes towards women's education are still confused. Although boys and girls are equally entitled to formal education and are generally thought to be equally capable of benefiting from it, teachers, parents and children believe that it is less necessary for girls. This attitude is closely connected with the expectation that qualifications, a job and a career are less important for women who will probably work full time only while they are waiting to marry, and whose lives shortly after marriage will be focused primarily on their families rather than on paid employment. This is the beginning of the vicious circle. Not helped to think much beyond marriage and the rearing of children, girls find numerous pressures on them to fit in with the common stereotype of a woman's role. For many women who become disenchanted with this role one of these pressures is their limited educational qualifications.

Although there have in recent years been significant changes in attitudes towards men and women's place in society, and therefore towards their education, these still reflect beliefs about sharp divisions between male and female roles. Indeed, there is some evidence that these beliefs are so deep rooted that they are not easily affected by deliberate educational efforts. When great attention has been paid to minimising the differences between the formal socialisation and education of boys and girls, mothers who were convinced of the importance of these efforts still found it difficult to support them fully in practice; their expectations of their daughters and the way they treated them continued to reflect traditional notions about the abilities, duties and lot of women (Dahlstrom, 1967). Gavron (1968) found in her study of housewives that even among those who were discontented with their confined and domestic lives, a significant number thought education less important for girls than for boys. This seemed to reflect a belief in the inevitability and permanence of some of the constraints in a woman's life and a resignation to them. Studies of child rearing have shown that although *within* the family male and female roles have become considerably more flexible during the last two generations, boys and girls are left in no doubt that their futures will be very different. From earliest childhood there are expectations that they will, in certain respects, behave in ways traditionally regarded as either masculine or feminine. One of the most obvious examples of these expectations can be seen in children's play and in the books they read. It is common for girls to be given toys which reflect the traditional female activities of the care of children, housekeeping, cooking and sewing while boys are expected to enjoy sport and playing with constructional toys. Children's books also frequently portray girls' interests as being primarily domestic, whereas boys are seen as being more involved outside the home and in leadership roles (Parsons and Bales, 1964; Young and Wilmott, 1957; J. and E. Newson, 1965 and 1970; Oakley, 1974a).

In short, it is women's biological role as mothers, although limited in time, which is the strongest influence in their upbringing. To a large extent women's status in society derives from their ascribed destiny as wives and mothers, whereas the status of men tends to be 'achieved' in that it depends on what they do and the work they perform. Since it is commonly assumed that existing institutions are both right and unchangeable it is all too easy for a self-perpetuating culture to develop in which a woman's main, albeit brief, role is maternal.

Some sobering facts illustrate the trends that have been described. Even though there are more girls than boys in the upper streams of mixed schools, fewer girls than boys sit school-leaving examinations, especially the higher level examinations that are required for universities and polytechnics. A girl's chances of going to a university, compared with those of a man, are poorer than they were fifty years ago. More girls than boys leave school at the earliest age and there is some evidence that girls do less well than they are able because they fear that academic success will lessen their chances of being viewed as acceptable girlfriends and wives. There are fewer training schemes and apprenticeships for girls and far fewer receive any form of further education. Provision for the technical education of girls is sparse and the subjects they most commonly study tend to fit them for traditional female roles. They therefore lack the qualifications necessary for a very large number of jobs including those associated with rapid technological expansion (Select Committee on Anti-Discrimination, 1973).

In general, therefore, it would be fair to say that parents and schools have failed to help girls to plan for a long and varied life in which the full-time upbringing of children will occupy only a third of their adult years. There is also insufficient guidance about the choice of jobs which will allow women to have a dual commitment to her work and her home. For example, clerical and office work, the traditional goals of vast numbers of unmarried female employees, are frequently incompatible with married women's needs for part-time work or work with flexible hours and reasonable holidays.

Several problems face those in a position to influence young girls' choice of occupation. The most difficult is helping the individual balance the current realities of the job market with her own aspirations and strengths, while holding onto the fact that the conditions of female employment are changing, and will change more radically, partly in response to women's contribution and to their demands for equal treatment.

At its most bleak the choice may be between an occupation which is compatible with fairly traditional definitions of marriage and motherhood, but which may have inherent disadvantages, and one which may have instrinsic satisfactions for the woman concerned but be extremely difficult to combine with her domestic responsibilities. The latter option has much to commend it in terms of independence and challenge to traditional divisions of employment along sex lines. But the costs of such a choice may be considerable if it means conflict and strain for a woman whose decision to work is not supported by her family and who receives little help with her other responsibilities. Limited achievement at home and at work can lead to frustration and feelings of failure.

To help her make her decision a girl needs full information about the conditions and implications of different kinds of employment, a chance to consider her own strengths and potential and the support she would be willing to use and likely to receive. She also needs to think how she would like her life to develop during the half century and more which is before her when she leaves school. With such opportunities often lacking women's decisions are frequently haphazard and unpremeditated.

Decisions about employment cannot be separated from an understanding of the roles of men and women and the responsibilities of parenthood. Discussion of such matters should be a part of courses in human relationships and sex education which, even if they exist at all, are often limited in their scope. Opportunities for boys to learn about child care and household tasks are also important if they are later to be able, naturally and easily, to share domestic responsibilities with their wives, so making it practically possible for both of them to lead lives in which there is no exclusive commitment either to home or to work.

That this flexibility already exists is apparent from several research studies and leads some to be optimistic about the future shape of women's lives. Nevertheless, greater sharing between men and women usually grows from the recognition of the strains on many housewives, especially the mothers of young children. It has not often been anticipated as a natural part of married life and parenthood. This would be more common if young women, and therefore by implication their boyfriends and husbands, were accustomed to take a long view of their lives which would set in its proper perspective that part likely to be dominated by motherhood.

The following extract from a letter written by a young mother to her former teacher reveals very clearly the feelings of many women that they have not been helped to think of themselves as other than wives and mothers.

You will probably have heard about the arrival of our third child. Perhaps you will remember that I always thought two would be the ideal number. However, as I saw that James and Anne, who will soon be at school, seemed to need much less of my attention, I began to wonder how I might fill the time. I toyed with the idea of going back to work. As you know I loved my job as a secretary. But I thought it would probably be difficult to find work with the right hours; even more, I wondered if I could still manage the various skills necessary. I have been at home so much that I don't have a great deal of confidence in the way I would cope with a job outside. I know that John would have helped me with the children but he didn't seem very keen on the idea of my working. In fact he seemed very surprised that I should want to do anything outside our very nice home. My mum seemed a bit shocked too and scared me with stories of children who had started to behave badly and steal because their mothers worked. And so without really thinking about it too much the best thing seemed to be another baby. This would give me a proper reason for staying at home and everyone seemed to think it was a good idea.

Michael is really sweet, and I love him very much, but I must be honest and say I wonder what I shall do when he goes to school. I will only be thirty-four then but I can't go on having a string of babies. I think it will be even more difficult to go back to work then than it seemed last year. I sometimes feel very angry that I didn't have the chance to think all this out before. I often long for some of the ordinary satisfactions and independence of work and am bored by much of the 'sameness' of being at home. I'm afraid this sometimes makes me a pretty resentful wife and mum. I can be shocking to live with. What frightens me most at the moment is wondering how I shall sort out my life when the children are older . . . .

Women's self-perceptions: masculinity and femininity

Are we dealing with a must that we dare not flout because it is rooted so deep in our biological mammalian nature that to flout it means individual and social disaster? Or with a must that, although not so deeply rooted, still is so very socially convenient and so well tried that it would be uneconomical to flout it – a must which says, for example, that it is easier to get children born and bred if we stylise the behaviour of the sexes very differently, teaching them to walk and dress and act in contrasting ways and to specialise in different kinds of work (Mead, 1954a, pp. 17-18).

Much of the argument about the appropriate education and employment of women rests on assumptions about the attributes of masculinity and femininity. These assumptions greatly influence perceptions of the needs, capabilities and duties of both sexes and they are often advanced as justifications for the differences in their responsibilities and treatment. In short, it is argued men and women's natures determine existing social arrangements.

For centuries members of different disciplines have attempted to define and explain the various personality and behaviour traits which have, at different times, been thought to be linked to sex.

During the last hundred years, with the development of the social sciences and the movement for the emancipation of women, this subject has received renewed attention. There has been much dispute among anthropologists, psychologists and sociologists, to mention only a few of the interested parties, about their respective findings and conclusions, many of which seem today to be extraordinarily superficial (Klein, 1946). In general, the task of identifying traits of personality or behaviour which could be described as particularly masculine or feminine has proved to be a fruitless one. Historians and anthropologists have shown conclusively that behaviour which may be the prerogative of women in one culture or in one epoch, may be the prerogative of men in others (Mead, 1954a; Oakley, 1974a). Nevertheless, in any particular society it does seem possible to identify types of behaviour which are associated more with one sex than the other. These characteristics are not primarily the result of anatomical or constitutional differences but largely the consequences of socialisation processes designed to prepare men and women for different social roles (Hutt, 1972; Oakley, 1972).

Although it is sometimes argued that there are inherent psychological differences between men and women, psychologists have concluded that the personality traits labelled as masculine and feminine are present to some extent in both sexes. In other words, men and women have both masculine and feminine aspects of their personalities, although for various reasons both tend to repress those characteristics generally held to be the prerogative of the opposite sex. Rapid social change, which is associated with increasingly flexible expectations of the roles of men and women, will mean constantly shifting definitions of masculinity and femininity and a growing acceptance that behaviour and personality need not conform to rigid stereotypes. These changes will affect some groups more quickly than others and there will probably continue to be differences between the social classes about what passes as acceptable conduct.

Some common stereotypes

What characteristics tend today to be seen as primarily masculine and feminine? And what criticisms are there of these definitions? Parsons (1964) has provided one of the best-known analyses of masculine and feminine behaviour. He distinguished two types of role within the family. The instrumental role involves dealing with external contingencies and the relationship of the family to society; it therefore entails accomplishment in the wider social world and calls for qualities of leadership, organisation and decision-making. The expressive role concerns the maintenance of the family as a unit, the promotion of good relationships between individuals and the reduction of stress. Parsons observed that the instrumental role is performed largely by the husband and the expressive by the wife. The qualities each needs to accomplish his or her allotted role tend to reflect traditional Western perceptions of male and female characteristics. Men are required to be ambitious, outgoing and primarily occupied with affairs outside the family; by contrast women are said to be more passive, more concerned with the emotional aspects of life and the promotion and maintenance of close family relationships, and less involved with the outside world. Many people would now be suspicious of such generalisations. Parsons himself acknowledged that there would be shifts of emphasis in these roles and was well aware that a woman's family responsibilities demanded some 'instrumental' qualities. Nevertheless, whatever changes may be taking place, this analysis still seems to be consistent with some common perceptions of a woman's role.

The image, even when humorous and caricatured, of the man's hard day's work and the woman's preoccupation with domestic concerns in the promotion of the happiness of her husband and offspring is a familiar one. Every variety writer knows that he will be able to raise a knowing laugh by portraying this same woman's silliness and ineptness at traditionally 'masculine' tasks. Women's magazines continue to publish articles describing appropriate strategies for attracting men. These include always allowing them to appear cleverer than women and to make all the important decisions. The content of television commercials are further evidence of the lack of surprise or outrage with images of women as irrational, emotional, passive creatures whose chief interests are babies and the embellishment of their homes, and whose chief assets are their looks and sweet natures.

We do not know how large is the gap between these unsubtle stereotypes and men and women's actual perceptions of female characteristics. Increasing flexibility in social roles probably means that it is widening, although the fact that such stereotypes have any currency is in itself significant. That they do have some influence is evident from the attitudes to the education of women which have already been described. In so far as girls are helped to think at all about their long-term futures it seems that many, particularly those in the lower social groups, are subjected to double standards. Myrdal and Klein (1968) suggest that throughout their education young women are likely to be vulnerable to one of the basic conflicts inherent in Western culture, which at one and the same time fosters individual assertion and competitiveness while also making much of the Christian virtues of love between neighbours and the suppression of selfish desires. While girls are persuaded that a boyfriend and husband will best be won by a show of sweetness, submission, dependence and limited aspirations, common sense tells them that once they have children they will need to be good managers, resourceful, organised and, especially if they work, adept at meeting a number of different demands on their time and personality. It is therefore not surprising that many girls are confused about which aspects of their personalities they should present and cultivate.

Women in society; some beliefs and questions

These short accounts of women at home, at school and at work raise many questions about their and, therefore by implication, men's proper social roles. Few subjects have aroused more heat and irrationality, or have been so obscured by a confusion of facts and ideology. The long debate engendered the greatest passions some seventy years ago with the struggles of the suffragettes for emancipation. With the achievements of the main objectives of the suffragettes' campaign, it seemed at first as if women had only to enjoy the fruits of their success. Recent years have seen a revival of concern about women's position in society (de Beauvoir, 1953; Rossi, 1965 and 1973; Figes, 1970; Greer, 1971; Millett, 1971). While it is probably true that contemporary social attitudes are now much more flexible and informed, the notion that women should make full use of the opportunities which exist, and that there should be further reforms to ensure less differentiated and ascribed social roles, still meets with more ambivalence and hostility than enthusiasm. The usually confused argument about the liberation of women, in its frequent trivialisation of important issues, reveals a lack of understanding of the nature and origin of much of the discontent in women's lives.

Nevertheless, it is not surprising that the arguments about

women's contemporary roles should prove threatening. In their examination of the influence of various social institutions, including the organisation of family life, they challenge long established conventional understanding of the nature of women and of the social order. They show how supposed differences between the sexes, and the inequalities for women that proceed from these suppositions, are the consequence, not the cause, of women's economic dependence and the limited social roles which accompany this. It follows therefore that at the very least, significant changes in the position of women can only come about with a radical transformation of attitudes and aspirations and a reordering of roles and responsibilities within existing social structures. From a more revolutionary standpoint, others argue that these changes could only come to pass in a society not dominated by traditional notions of family life.

It is also uncomfortable when parallels are drawn between the position of women and that of other underprivileged groups, such as ethnic minorities. Both may be seen as only capable of filling certain roles in society; both are discriminated against and both suffer from economic and educational deprivation (Mitchell, 1971).

Analyses such as these are helpful in that they force us not to focus narrowly on the position of women but to relate the existence of inequality and underprivilege to the economic and social organisation of societies in which power is unevenly distributed. In a capitalist economy there is a strong tendency for power and status to belong to the economically productive. One consequence is that despite their often poor conditions of work, it is to women's advantage to be paid employees as well as wives and mothers.

It might be argued that, to the extent that women are not expected to endure the burdens of continuous membership of the labour force, they are in a privileged position. This view rests largely on the assumption that the intrinsic satisfactions of motherhood and domestic life preclude the necessity of any financial reward, an assumption which is not extended to those men who find intrinsic satisfactions in their work. It seems as if women, in direct contradiction to prevailing beliefs and social conditions which associate economic power with notions of 'the good life', are charged with the responsibility of proving that, after all, material gain and its associated privileges are not the highest goals of society.

Challenges to such a comforting belief are difficult to make and strongly resisted. They are, however, increasingly likely as women, in flight from the isolation and constraints of the nuclear family, taste the rewards of employment outside the home. It is also arguable that, as men and women come to experience both the pains and pleasures of paid employment and domestic life, they increasingly seek a life with opportunities for a reasonable division between the two. Many women have already opted for such a life, and with ever-decreasing working hours, this also becomes a possibility for men (Williams, 1969; Halsey, 1972a). Such an arrangement seems to allow the fullest expression of men and women's interests and potential and challenges the now rapidly dating assumptions about differences in masculine and feminine capabilities and aspirations. Opportunities for a more equal division in the labour of men and women need not mean a worse life for the former, although a better one for the latter, but an improvement in the quality of life of both.

What does this brief discussion of the changing position of women in society as mothers and wives have to contribute to an understanding of attitudes to pregnancy and child rearing? Mitchell (1971) provides an answer to this question in her analysis of women's position in terms of four dimensions. These are the productive, reproductive and socialisation systems of society and the arrangements for sanctioning sexual bonds. In Western societies these last three processes find expression in the family, which provides the context for continuing sexual relationships between men and women and for the rearing of children. Mitchell discusses the relationships between these systems and shows how the position of women in different societies and at different times can be explained in terms of alterations in these relationships. We have already seen how recent changes in the economic productive system of society have had a profound influence on the structure of family life. However, Mitchell goes on to argue convincingly that changes in any one of these four systems will not radically influence the position of women unless they are accompanied by changes in the other three. For example, the political enfranchisement of women, when not accompanied by fundamental changes in the educational or socialisation systems and in the economic situation, accomplished far less than originally had been hoped or feared. Additionally, efforts to reduce inequalities in employment which are based on sex, if they are to be successful, must be accompanied by changes in education, social security and taxation and in provision for the substitute care of children. Recent British legislation allows for only some of these changes.

It is also possible for a modification in the demands of any one system to be offset by an increase in those of another. Although women today spend far fewer years than their forebears in the upbringing of young children, changing ideas about their needs and rising expectations of desired standards of child care mean that there are now pressures on mothers to devote themselves almost entirely to this. One consequence is that more care is lavished on fewer children. Whatever the merits of this situation, and these will be discussed later, it still requires seeing the prime function of women as motherhood.

These complex relationships between various social institutions and the position of women mean that the partial changes which have occurred in family patterns, education and employment may be the source of frustration as well as opportunity, especially if prevailing customs and social arrangements force a woman to choose between a life dominated primarily by domestic or by work responsibilities. Expectations rise before the means of fulfilling them has been found.

In such a situation it is inevitable that many women will feel ambivalent about the costs and gains of their roles as mothers. Paradoxically, the fact that pregnancy can be avoided adds to this uncertainty because no longer can women argue generally that their fates have largely been thrust upon them. They cannot escape making some choice about their lives or experiencing the uncertainty and regrets that are the price of independence. These dilemmas may well contribute to the widespread haphazard, sporadic and apparently 'irrational' use of contraception noticed by Cartwright (1970) and Bone (1973).

Women and their children

It may be objected that the picture so far drawn of a woman's life is a dismal one which makes little allowance for the deep satisfactions and pleasures of marriage and motherhood. Have not the risks of discontent been exaggerated? Do not the differences between the social classes and between individuals mean that it is impossible to generalise about women's reactions? This section will attempt to answer these questions but it must immediately be admitted that there are no reliable methods of assessing the happiness or discontent of half the population. We are largely dependent on symptoms of social and emotional distress and interpretations of the likely consequences of certain aspects of our society. We also have to weigh the shortcomings and disadvantages of earlier social arrangements and take into account existing health and welfare provisions. Most importantly, we have to learn to accept the paradox that the greater seem to be the possibilities of achieving happiness, the more choices there are before people, and the higher their aspirations, the greater too are the chances of discontent and disappointment.

The social context of child rearing

The social cult of maternity is matched only by the socio-economic powerlessness of the mother (Mitchell, 1971, p. 109).

What is known about women's reactions to the period of their lives which is dominated by child rearing? To some extent the care of young children has become easier. Various health and welfare provisions protect their physical well-being, and although large numbers of families still live in great poverty and appalling housing conditions, the majority are reasonably economically secure. Against this, pressures to keep up with the standards of an affluent society mean that many people become discontented with a style of life which seems to mark them out as relative failures. Determination to improve this situation is one factor which prompts mothers to work.

These consequences of a capitalist economy have other costs. The separation of young parents from their relatives means that mothers are more isolated today than ever before. The kind of accommodation which accompanies rapid urban development also increases this isolation when it involves living on housing estates on the edge of towns and away from ordinary social amenities, or in high-rise flats which make it difficult to cultivate relationships with neighbours. Lack of play space near such accommodation means that young children cannot be left by their mothers to play independently. They may therefore never be apart from each other. Few women, or their children, can tolerate living at such close quarters with equanimity.

These difficulties have arisen at the same time as the developments in knowledge about the emotional needs of young children. Most parents now know that it is widely accepted that their infants need the security which will come from the regular and consistent care which is usually provided by a child's mother or close relatives. Parents are also anxious to help their young children to develop socially and intellectually by providing suitable opportunities for play. The rapid development of pre-school playgroups is evidence of these new concerns.

In most families it is mothers who carry the main responsibility for meeting these high standards of child care. Not all of them feel equipped for this. Paradoxically, although girls' education assumes their eventual motherhood, it does not usually involve much preparation for the care of young children, except perhaps for their most basic physical needs. Mothercraft classes for pregnant women are also largely concerned with the care of very young babies and although the need for preparation for parenthood is now recognised, it has not yet become much more than a slogan. Moreover, these strains usually fall on women at a time when they are economically totally dependent and socially isolated.

Domestic satisfactions

The invention of many household appliances and the mass production of prepared foods have reduced much of the drudgery that used to be the normal lot of the housewife. Such time-saving devices, which have made it easier for women to go out to work, have also been accompanied by a movement to raise the standards of cooking and household care and to bring back into the home activities which used to be performed by outside agencies. The Do-It-Yourself industry, whether concerned with home decorating, brewing, baking or the making of clothes, is not only popular because of its obvious economies but because performing these tasks can be the source of real satisfaction. This seems to be particularly true for women if the huge sales of the relevant magazines and materials can be taken as evidence. Not surprisingly, since accomplishment in these new 'home industries' means added comforts and luxuries, they are likely to receive support from husbands and children. No doubt the hours they involve largely account for the findings of Myrdal and Klein (1968) and Friedan (1971) that the household duties of mothers who did not go out to work took up nearly as many hours as those of the women who did.

It is all too easy in this debate to adopt a moralising position about what women should or should not enjoy. The satisfaction derived from tasks which others think unnecessary is still satisfaction. Undoubtedly many women are completely content to occupy themselves totally in the care of their families. These women may, however, face a crisis when their children leave home if they feel deprived of their function in life. Others may be less satisfied with total domestic preoccupation but be prepared to commit themselves to this, and make the best of it, for a period of their lives. Nevertheless, evidence is accumulating which shows that women who make this commitment either from choice or necessity do not envisage it as involving the care of several children over a long period.

Married women and unwanted pregnancies

Although various studies have revealed a high rate of unplanned and unwanted pregnancy amongst married women these studies also show that many women are pleased when they become pregnant even when they have been taking precautions to prevent this. There are some women too who, although they have apparently decided to have no more children, are deliberately careless in their use of contraception and pleased with the resulting 'accidents'. Such behaviour and reactions show just how complex are women's attitudes to child bearing. There are certainly some women whose pleasure in motherhood seems to undermine their decisions and actions to prevent pregnancy.

There remain, however, a large number of women for whom the arrival of one more pregnancy is definitely an unwelcome event. The fact that such pregnancies will frequently mean that the family remains small, and the time spent in the care of children only slightly extended, does not appear to make them welcome, as is evident from Bone's and Cartwright's studies and from the large numbers of young married women with two or three children who ask for abortions. Despite the use of more effective contraception between 1966 and 1973 Cartwright (1976) found there was no change in the proportion of legitimate births which were initially unwanted. As parents' expectations about their ability to control pregnancies grow their toleration of unintended pregnancies appears to diminish.

This dismay at unintended pregnancy also has to be understood in the context of the intended family size of married couples. Woolf's study (1971) of this most complex subject illustrates the connection between an appreciation of financial and material pressures and intentions to have small families. Although a substantial proportion of women believed that three or four children was the ideal number for families with no money worries, half of them said that their own circumstances made two children the most desirable number. This wish for small families was particularly evident among working-class couples married during the early 1960s. On the basis of information about the reported contraceptive practice (but not of the various failures and problems in the use of contraception). Woolf concluded that expectations with regard to family size were likely to be borne out in reality, especially for women married after 1959. In recent years the number of children couples want at the time of their marriage appears to have declined still further (Cartwright, 1976).

Such studies confirm that women, increasingly aware of the options before them, wish to play an active part in shaping the destinies of their families. They are not happily deflected from their purpose.

The mothers speak

If the trends which have been described throw some light on the possible attitudes of women towards their domestic life and the care of their children, what more can these women tell us themselves? Although it is usually more likely that studies will note the existence of problems than success, and of discontent than delight, a few studies have made careful attempts to obtain a broad picture of the lives of mothers from different social classes and the upbringing of their children (J. and E. Newson, 1965 and 1970; Gavron, 1968). Friedan's (1971) study of American housewives is more anecdotal but makes interesting observations on the outlook of middle-class mothers, as does the Rapoports' (1971) study of dual-career families.

These researches all provide good illustrations, in personal terms, of the impact of motherhood on women in contemporary society. They confirm that most mothers find the care of their children, particularly when they are babies, imposes greater strains than they had expected. They also feel ignorant and incompetent. Gavron remarks (1968, p. 79):

> The lives of these young mothers centred around their children and their home. There were indications that they were not fully prepared for the responsibilities of motherhood imposed on them and many were acutely aware of the restrictions it imposed on their lives. But their response to this, in the majority of cases, was to take the responsibility of motherhood very seriously and to devote to it much serious thought.

This feeling that children's futures rest largely in their mothers' hands is reflected in the comment of one of the mothers in the Newsons' first study (1965, p. 258):

> Nowadays if they don't turn out right you wonder where you've gone wrong, don't you? It used to be, they made you do this and do that and you did it and if things went wrong it was the child's fault not the parents'; they could never be wrong. I think we are not so happy about ourselves these days, we blame ourselves, not the child.

Freedom from passive acceptance of traditional wisdom about child care brings with it not only the pleasures of independence but also the strain of making decisions and the pain of responsibility for mistakes made.

The majority of mothers in these studies did not carry these burdens alone; a high proportion of their husbands participated actively in the running of the home and the care of children. Although this help was much appreciated many of the wives rightly remarked that it did not alter the fact that they were on their own with their children for the major part of the day (Oakley, 1974b). While their husbands moved in two worlds, they moved in only one. For working-class women particularly, this sense of isolation was exacerbated by limited social contacts. Contrary to widespread assumptions Gavron found parents' focus of interest to be on the nuclear rather than the extended family. Many women who had moved to unfamiliar neighbourhoods also lacked the confidence and social skills necessary to make new friends. They were therefore almost entirely dependent on their husbands for companionship. There was also either a lack or distrust of facilities for the temporary substitute care of children which would make it possible for parents to have some social life of their own.

> It appears that the period when children are young is for many working class couples one of isolation and withdrawal into the home during which time the main contact with the outside world is via the television (Gavron, 1968, p.100).

Middle-class mothers

If these experiences are reasonably common for all mothers of young children, do middle- and working-class women have their own particular problems? The Newsons thought that for many middle-class women the arrival of young children could be especially traumatic. More than her working-class sisters a middle-class woman has been educated to think of herself as an independent person in her own right. She may therefore find the presence of young children, especially if this means giving up all idea of work, frustrates her from fulfilling what she considers to be her rightful role.

> Many middle class mothers seem to see the period of infancy in particular not as time of fulfilment, but as an abnormal and in many ways deplorable interlude in an otherwise sane and well ordered life . . . . Such a woman finds it difficult to reconcile her ideal self image as a mature sophisticated woman with her roles as a housebound baby minde;, nappy washer and domestic slave (J. and E. Newson, 1965, p. 223).

The Rapoports (1971) remark that the shock and frustration felt with the arrival of a first baby are especially acute for women who are deeply involved in their careers and wish to continue to work. Even when these women have planned their babies they are often ambivalent about motherhood and for them the arrival of their first child may precipitate a crisis of personal identity.

> It is not only mental concentration that is sapped by baby care and housework, it is personality concentration as well. A baby

demands the whole of you. Before I had him I could turn away
from everybody into myself or my books if I needed to . . . .
But I remain turned towards Carl even when he is asleep.
At first this was a terrible burden. Now I bear it lightly
(Fraser, 1968, p. 146).

These difficulties are to some extent offset by middle-class
women's ability to arrange an active social life, to organise part-
time work and to see this period of relative frustration as a
temporary phase to be tolerated and lived through. The rather sad
observations of the Newsons that many middle-class mothers
seemed to live nostalgically in the past remembering early adult
life as a time of gay adventure and unfettered freedom and that
they were not, openly at least, much enjoying their children's
babyhood, may reflect the dilemmas of women who doubt
whether they can combine the roles of mother and worker, and are
despondent at the prospect of a primarily domestic life.

Despite these difficulties these mothers seem to be in a happier
position than the American women studied by Friedan (1971) who
appeared overwhelmed by the prospect of apparently unending
motherhood. Many of these often highly educated middle-class
women had married young, partly because they were frightened of
the social consequences of committing themselves to careers. Once
they became mothers they seemed to lose confidence in their
ability ever again to work outside their homes. Most of these
women said they lived vicariously through their husbands and
children, and most resented this deeply.

Working-class mothers

A working-class woman's problems may be rather different.
Although she is more likely to have been brought up to see
motherhood as her destiny and to expect her fulfilment and social
status to derive from this, there are many pressures which make it
difficult for her to enjoy this role. First, her comparative isolation
means that there are few people with whom she can share the
pleasures and trials of motherhood. Her world is thus far more
limited than she had imagined. Gavron thought these mothers
especially likely to be victims of the sense of confusion and let
down which arises when women are led to regard marriage as a
kind of unending affair in which the partners are expected to

remain at the high point of infatuation for the rest of their lives. Added to these disappointments are frequent economic and material problems. Overwhelmed by poor housing, limited play facilities and a low income, many working-class women could see no end to this difficult period in their lives.

Attitudes towards children

Lest it should be thought that these researchers paint an unreal picture of unrelieved gloom it must be emphasised that most of the children in the families studied were loved and wanted, and the source of much pleasure and satisfaction.

The Newsons' study of four-year-olds reveals especially a deep reservoir of tenderness for children of this age and, when these were the last children, about to go to school, the regret of many mothers that one phase of their life was over, however demanding it had been. Studies of older children also show that although parents continue their self-conscious efforts to understand their offspring and bring them up well, and are still vulnerable to feelings of failure, the passing years give them greater confidence in their abilities. Most parents are also determined to have fun with their children and to enjoy them as friends and companions. They are, however, aware of the strains, as well as the pleasures, of this relationship of relative equality. It is not always easy to accept the more spirited, disrespectful child who is the result of a relaxed and permissive approach to upbringing. This relationship of studied ease may require a very special kind of commitment and resilience.

A particular compensation for the more limited horizons of a working-class woman is the high status which may be allotted to her as 'our mum' (Bott, 1957; Klein, 1965; J. and E. Newson, 1965 and 1970). To be the one person on whom the whole household depends can be highly satisfying and the children of such a woman are often viewed as her proud possession, a symbol of status in themselves and an extension to her own personality. These rewards often seem to outweigh the strains of motherhood.

Bearing in mind these obvious pleasures of caring for children, one of the most interesting facts to emerge from Gavron's work concerns the high proportion of mothers who would like to work if circumstances permitted. There is no reason to suppose that these mothers were any less attached to their children than the

Newson mothers (who were not asked about their future work plans), but about 70 per cent still said they would like to be at work, at least part time. However, in most cases this wish conflicted with their sense of responsibility as mothers. Mothers either felt it would be wrong to leave their young children regularly in the care of anyone else, or that it would be impossible to make adequate arrangements for their alternative care. For most mothers paid employment is only feasible if they can be sure of the highest standards of care for their children (R. and R. N. Rapoport, 1971).

It is possible that the fears of mothers about the implications of temporary alternative care for children are not always well founded. Evidence from research studies relating to the separation of children from their mothers is frequently misinterpreted and some gross generalisations are made (chapter 6). Nevertheless, there is an absolute shortage of good day care, and in the absence of reasonable alternatives to staying at home there will be pressures for existing arrangements to be seen as the best.

Whatever the reasons for most mothers' convictions that they should stay at home when their children are small, nearly all the women Gavron studied were planning to work when their children were older and were looking forward to this. There was little difference in this respect between middle-class and working-class women; the latter were just as eager to return to work despite lack of education and training and limited employment opportunities. The remark of one of these mothers expresses the prevailing feeling that the rewards of a totally home-bound life, real though these could be, are insufficient. 'Measured by the values of a society like this where the real business of life is held to be what people do during their working hours, I'm standing still. I don't exist, (Gavron, 1968, p. 132).

This account of inequalities and discontents is disturbing. Although not true for all women, they are more common than we have been prepared to admit, and it would be more comfortable to deny or make light of them. They are problems intimately connected with women's roles as mothers and a future which too often seems a muddle of irreconcilable alternatives. For women's sake, and the sake of their families, these problems deserve serious examination. And ways must be found of creating a better balance between the pleasures and fulfilment and the vicissitudes of parenthood.

three

Psychological insights

The longevity of the oppression of women *must* be based on something more than conspiracy, something more complicated than biological handicap and more durable than economic exploitation. It is illusory to see women as the pure who are purely put upon: the status of women is held in the heart and the head as well as the home: oppression has not been trivial or historically transitory – to maintain itself so effectively it courses through the mental and emotional bloodstream (Mitchell, 1974, p. 362).

The most important data about people are not their vital statistics but those relating to their hopes and fears, loves and hates, satisfactions and frustrations and to companionship and loneliness (Venables, 1971, p. 3).

Emotional problems of childbearing are not separate and isolated – related only to having babies. They are an integral part of the fact of being a woman (Kitzinger, 1962, p. 42).

The previous chapter's brief account of the social changes and pressures which influence women's lives is crucial to an understanding of their problems but, as the quotations from Mitchell and Venables imply, necessary generalisations about social trends cannot, on their own, explain any individual woman's experience of pregnancy and motherhood. For her, and for those who try to help her, what is held 'in the heart and the head' is of greater significance than the various social and economic forces which, in isolation, will probably appear remote and abstract.

Psychological insights can therefore contribute greatly to the understanding of an individual woman's experiences, and this chapter outlines briefly those which are particularly relevant to pregnancy, childbirth and motherhood.

There is not a very large literature on which to draw and what there is falls into two main divisions, although there is considerable overlap between them. The first consists largely of the work of psychiatrists and clinical psychologists who have interested themselves in the emotional changes which are said to characterise pregnancy and the puerperium. Then there is the work of psychoanalysts and those who have drawn on their insights without accepting all their conclusions. Their most valuable contribution for counsellors is a view of pregnancy and early motherhood not as hurdles to be overcome, so that a woman may return to her normal equilibrium, but as a stage of development, as events which set in motion interacting social and emotional processes, with influences for good or ill.

Emotional reactions to pregnancy

In the year or so between conception and an infant's first few months of life extreme swings of mood are common. The first three months of pregnancy are often described as a period of heightened emotional sensitivity, of elation and depression, of irritability and aggression (Caplan, 1961; Baker, 1967; Kaig and Nilsson, 1972; and Horobin et al., 1973).

No certain predictions about a woman's eventual adjustment to motherhood can be made on the basis of these early reactions. Some women who are at first horrified by their pregnancies eventually accept them happily and appear to cope successfully with motherhood (Breen, 1975). Others who may joyfully accept pregnancy as a resolution to unsolved problems of identity may be bitterly disappointed to find that motherhood merely delays rather than provides an answer to this question. Only for a very limited part of her total life span can a woman state 'I do not have to be anything because I am pregnant' (Deutsch, 1946). Once again we see the importance of flexible definitions of 'unwanted pregnancy'.

The second three months of pregnancy are often more peaceful with women becoming more introverted and passive. This is followed in the last trimester by periods of restlessness and anxiety, even panic, as women come ever closer to a meeting between their fantasies and the reality of their infants and of themselves as mothers. These preoccupations may continue for some weeks after delivery (Lomas, 1967).

It seems, therefore, that during pregnancy women tend to be more than usually in touch with their feelings and with memories of their childhood. This is a time when forgotten conflicts and problems come to the fore. These may be the relics of old struggles about a woman's identity, the clashes between the person she wanted to be and the person she felt obliged to become, or of her ambivalent feelings towards her parents, brothers and sisters. Although some of this heightened sensitivity and emotional lability is almost certainly connected with physiological changes which accompany pregnancy, there are other significant factors.

First, both planned and unplanned pregnancies may be accompanied by financial worries and the problems of finding accommodation suitable for parents and children. Second, a pregnant woman can quite suddenly find herself swept into an exclusive culture of reproduction and motherhood which may be alien to her. It is a world in which she is often regarded as a passive object, whose sole responsibility is to impart highly personal information, submit to intimate examinations and follow unquestioningly the advice and directives of doctors and nurses. Lack of privacy and respect for a woman's individuality may continue through childbirth and after delivery, frequently allowing her little opportunity to be alone with and to get to know her baby (Kitzinger, 1962).

It is easy to forget these harsh realities in pointing to the improvements in medicine and social welfare which have vastly reduced the dangers and discomforts of pregnancy and childbirth. Whatever her domestic situation the pregnant woman is the focus of much attention. Special shops cater for her needs and those of her baby. The books, the classes and the professional and neighbourly advice which help prepare women for childbirth are all evidence of the high value society attaches to the proper care of infants and their mothers. This welcome emphasis on the pleasures and privileges of motherhood nevertheless has its risks if it assumes pregnancy to be only a time of joyful anticipation, and the weeks after delivery a period of blissful fulfilment, marred only occasionally by a few days of depression. The paradox is that the very state which is expected to yield so much also makes great demands on the mother's physical and emotional energy, not least because it prompts a woman to reassess her past and future.

Identity, pregnancy and early motherhood

Pregnancy, particularly a first pregnancy, raises fundamental questions about a woman's identity. How will motherhood affect her status and her relationships with her husband and her parents?

Women who have worked, and enjoyed this, face the problem of relinquishing a role where their achievement is established for one which is unfamiliar and attracts little public acclaim. Older pregnant women may wonder about the implications of motherhood at a time when, with their other children's increasing independence, they might be expecting to re-establish themselves in employment. Alternatively, there may be anxieties about combining work and motherhood, anxieties which are often exacerbated by the prejudices of those who disapprove of working mothers. For the women who have always expected motherhood to endow them with status and to provide their main source of satisfaction there are fears about a possible gap between expectation and reality.

Pregnancy also means that a woman must start to reassess her closest relationships. What will it be like for her and her husband to share each other with a third, and initially very demanding and dependent person? What are her own parents' expectations of her as a mother? Will they share in their grandchildren's upbringing, or compete as rival influences? Have they provided a model of parenthood with which a woman can readily identify, even though she may not wish to reproduce it exactly? A woman whose chief memory of her mother is of a joyless drudge, given little support by her husband, and sharing little with him, can scarcely embark upon parenthood with confident anticipation. It is also unrealistic to focus on a woman's identification with her mother without also asking about her relationship with her father. The two must be closely linked. A woman's view of her femininity, her role in her new family and her relationship with men must be strongly influenced by these experiences.

Finally, and most crucially, how does a woman anticipate her responsibilities as a mother? Have her own experiences of family life left her confident that she can both give and receive love and tolerate the total dependence of an infant? Does she have the resources to establish a way of life which will meet her family's and her own needs. Deprived, resentful people cannot give much to others.

In short, pregnancy and motherhood prompt women to ask themselves what sort of people they are. In trying to answer this question they may well swing from joyfully seeing their pregnancy as providing them with a new reason for existence, and a new future, to fearing that they will not be equal to their children's demands and will be drained or eaten up by them (Deutsch, 1946). Such thoughts may be especially common towards the end of a pregnancy, when a woman's longing to have her baby in her arms may be accompanied by panic at the thought of an independent being whose separate existence, paradoxically, starts in a state of total dependence. This is also a time when women most commonly fear they will give birth to deformed children.

Most pregnant women ponder on these questions to which, until they have greater experience, they can produce no certain answers. And, as Caplan has remarked, it is dreams rather than reality which make us cowards. Most women want desperately to succeed as mothers but the price of this success may seem high and the conditions confusing. Such thoughts are echoed by the anxious mother who remarked that the ease of getting pregnant was matched only by the ease with which one could feel a failure as a mother. And there are many things which make women feel failures, including such transitory events as their perceptions of poor performances in giving birth, and their inadequacy in breast feeding. Winnicott, a psychiatrist who was much concerned with the interest of mothers and children, once remarked that it was now impossible to say or write anything about motherhood or the care of infants without making mothers feel guilty. This is one of the less happy results of the widespread acceptance of deeply self-conscious and responsible parenthood.

Resolving these problems

To be a mother equals to be like mother, to reject motherhood is to reject mother. Between these two extremes one may postulate various attempts at compromise (Kaig and Nilsson, 1972, p. 380).

How women resolve these questions of identity will depend on many factors, of which the most obvious is the support they receive from their husbands and close relatives and from various material and social resources. Less obvious, but in the opinion of many psychologists most important, is the image a woman has of her own mother, her identification with this image and her ability to be flexible in her expectations of herself as a mother. These memories and fantasies prompt the revival, and often the reassessment, of old problems. In the opinion of many workers it also provides a magnificent opportunity for emotional development, for the achievement of a comfortable sense of identity.

In a study of women's adaptation to the birth of their first child Breen (1975) found that their feelings of satisfaction were strongly related to their own positively valued experience of being mothered. Like other psychologists, Breen believes that a woman's capacity to value herself, and therefore to give love freely to other people, is rooted in this experience. Contrary to somewhat superficial assumptions that it is easy to love children, especially when they are young, the continual care of an infant makes the greatest demands on an individual, stirring the deepest feelings of love and hate.

In this study the women who adjusted least well were those who were preoccupied with somewhat rigid views of an ideal mother, views which seemed often to be linked to their own poor experience of mothering. These women were also pessimistic about their ability to achieve this goal, intolerant of their imperfections and prone to interpret everything they did as failure. Not surprisingly, they were particularly vulnerable to post-natal depression.

Amongst the better adjusted women there was no typical pattern. Some identified with a conventional definition of the mother's role; others reconstrued this to one they found personally comfortable. What they seemed to have in common was an ability to adapt their perception of motherhood, very often after the birth of their child, so as to minimise the conflict between their baby's demands, the pressures of their immediate environment, and their own needs. They seemed to have more open appraisals of themselves and other people and were thus able not to feel constrained by a narrow and largely unrealistic view of maternity. These women had been able to live up the assertion that,

In our civilisation, with its regulated births, woman has wide opportunities for making compromises between motherhood and her other, more personal needs, drives and interests. As a result there are as many variations in the psychology of motherhood as there are mothers (Deutsch, 1946, p. 259).

four

Parents and children with special difficulties

The fact itself of causing the existence of a human being is one
of the most responsible actions in the range of human life . . .
to bestow a life which may be either a curse or a blessing
– unless the being on whom it is to be bestowed will have at
least the ordinary chances of a desirable existence – is a
crime against that being (J. S. Mill, *On Liberty*, 1957, p. 163).

This chapter considers the problems of parents with particular
difficulties for whom the implications of an unwanted pregnancy
may be especially serious. These are frequently unsupported
women, the unmarried, the separated or divorced, or the very
young. Although the vicissitudes of these readily identifiable
groups are not *necessarily* greater than those of parents living in
more ordinary circumstances, numerous research studies provide
ample evidence of their special vulnerability. This must inevitably
increase risks of suffering for parents and children when a pregnancy is unwanted. What are these risks?

The consequences of unwanted pregnancy

It is difficult to give an exact answer to this question. The research
required to do this would be complex, demanding adequate
control groups, the continuation of the research over a number of
years and sensitive instruments of definition and measurement.
The difficulties of defining unwanted pregnancy are legion
(Chapter 1). While hard information can be obtained about a
family's composition, its income and housing, it is extremely
difficult to assess the quality of emotional and physical care given
to children, although it is this which crucially affects their
development.

We know that many unplanned, or initially unwanted, children come to be loved and accepted soon after birth. Others are tolerated with varying degrees of goodwill and some of these always feel partially rejected. Although it is often possible to identify children who are not fully accepted in their families, it is difficult to relate their situation to the circumstances of their mothers' pregnancies since there are also many such children whose births have been planned. It seems sensible therefore to accept that the degree to which children's births are welcomed is only one of a complex set of interrelated factors influencing their development (Illsley and Hall, 1975). It can, nevertheless, be of considerable importance, as is clear from studies of children born to mothers who have been refused an abortion.

The most well known of these studies and the one which followed up children over the longest period was carried out by Forssman and Thuwe (1966). Their study is a pioneering one, and although there have been some criticisms of its methodology and the control groups used, its conclusions are significant.

The researchers studied the mental health, social adjustment and educational level up to the age of twenty-one of 120 children born after their mothers' request for therapeutic abortion had been refused. They found that according to such criteria as the necessity for the child to be cared for outside his or her own home, complaints to official bodies about the care of the child, and the divorce of the parents, these children ran a greater risk of insecurity than did children in the control groups. They were also more likely to receive psychiatric treatment, to be reported for delinquent behaviour and to need some kind of public financial assistance. In addition, far more of the control children had some form of higher education. The authors conclude that the very fact that a woman seeks an authorised abortion, no matter how trivial her grounds may appear to be, means that the life chances of the expected child are likely to be poorer than those of other children.

Those who prefer to avoid termination of pregnancy wherever possible argue that it is far more constructive to give the parents and children concerned appropriate social and emotional help. There is not much evidence that a request for an abortion, certainly from a married couple, is the gateway to such assistance. Although social workers and others are often acutely aware of the problems associated with unwanted pregnancy, scarce resources mean only limited chances of help. This is confirmed by the studies of Horobin et al. (1973) of women requesting an abortion.

These researchers concluded that although the majority of women who continued their pregnancies eventually became reconciled to this, with most saying that they had positive feelings towards the child, the social and economic pressures on many of them, especially those in the lower social classes, gave rise to considerable concern.

> The suggestion that social support should be given as an alternative to abortion requested on primarily social grounds is not entirely realistic in the more chronic situations. Constructive help might entail rehousing a family, ensuring that a married woman has the security of some income under her control, seeing that maintenance grants are actually received or making far better provision for help with child care than at present exists. It is hardly necessary to say that denial of abortion does not entitle the over-burdened woman to special consideration of this kind and she is left to manage her increased family as best she can. It is as well to be clear about the reality of the 'social help' so easily invoked (p. 126).

Assistance is rather more likely to be forthcoming for unmarried girls. Even so, the help offered may be inadequate or inappropriate. For example, women who spend some time in homes for unmarried mothers and their infants may well suffer all kinds of privations, in a somewhat bleak environment, where compassion is tinged with sentimentality and treatment with punishment. The objectives of the care they receive may also be confused, ranging from efforts to help a girl set her pregnancy in the context of her life experiences and plan accordingly, to the simple offer of accommodation, with little other support (Nicholson, 1968).

For the single or unsupported mothers who keep their babies the help available is most inadequate (Wynn, 1964; Marsden, 1969; Holman, 1970 and 1975). Indeed, from a financial point of view, the most vulnerable children are those being brought up by single mothers. In 1974, 400,000 lone mothers were responsible for 720,000 children. Interestingly, the girl who marries as a result of her pregnancy is usually assumed, quite mistakenly, to have no further problems (Horobin et al., 1973).

To this list of reasonably well-documented problems can be added those which, although less researched, are the common knowledge of those who work with parents facing an unwanted pregnancy.

Not surprisingly, many women bearing an unwanted child are depressed during their pregnancies (Horobin *et al.*, 1973). As well as this depression there are anxieties about the practical difficulties of coping with the child and resentment against those thought to have contributed to the mother's dilemma. If these continue after the birth of the child the mother may find great difficulties with her baby. Problems with feeding and handling the child escalate when the response to inadequate care is incessant crying. Mothers in this situation are likely to feel double failures, believing their reactions towards their child to be unnatural, and thinking themselves incapable of decent maternal care.

Although some mothers and their children survive these early setbacks apparently unscarred there are others who are not so lucky. Most doctors, health visitors and social workers know several families where a child's maladjustment and his parents' consequent unhappiness can be related to an unwanted pregnancy. Research also suggests that mothers' inability to make a firm attachment to their young babies significantly affects their bonds with them in later childhood (Bowlby, 1969). Problems are also likely to ensue when the arrival of a child prevents the mother from pursuing interests of major importance to her, or when parents, whose relationship is crumbling, have sought but not been granted an abortion. It is also possible that parents who have been refused an abortion, and who have accepted their child, may subsequently feel guilty that they ever made such a request.

We do not yet know the extent of these problems, partly because they have only recently been acknowledged. Nevertheless, their gravity for the individuals concerned justifies giving special attention and help to parents faced with an unwanted pregnancy.

Parents and their natural children

The use of the word 'illegitimate' for children whose parents are not married can cause much distress and therefore, in accordance with the recommendation of the National Council of One Parent Families, the adjective 'natural' will be used instead.

During the past twenty years the number of natural children born has risen dramatically. Difficulties in obtaining divorce from former partners may be all that prevents the marriage of the parents of many of these children, although there are some for whom the formal bonds of marriage seem irrelevant (Parker, 1972). Probably about a third of all natural children now live in such families, but this proportion may decline because of the very large increase in illegitimate births to young single women who are unlikely to be living on a regular basis with the fathers of their children. Today the mothers of about two-thirds of the natural children born are under twenty-five, and a high proportion of these are aged between fifteen and nineteen.

There have also been other changes in the pattern of illegitimate births. Illegitimacy rates have fallen in rural but risen in urban areas, and illegitimate births are now more frequent than formerly among the upper socio-economic groups. Taken together these trends suggest,

> The emergence of a new pattern in the incidence of illegitimate birth associated with youth, urban living and sophistication at the very moment when an older pattern associated with rural life, poverty and family disorganisation was beginning to disappear (Illsley and Gill, 1968, p. 426).

The figures for illegitimate births to single women are, of course, no guide to the number of pregnancies occurring to them, since many of these end in abortion. In 1973 over 52,800 abortions were performed on single women (resident in England and Wales), and over 43,000 of these women were under twenty-five years of age. There are also large numbers of children born to parents who married after they had been conceived. There were about 67,000 of these pre-marital conceptions in 1971. If these births are added to the illegitimate ones, extra-marital conceptions now make up about 17 per cent of all live births.

The background to illegitimacy

> We need to think in terms of hypotheses to be truly tested rather than closed systems of explanation for which we are compelled to find substantiating evidence (Bernstein, 1966, p. 117).

> If we try to study why illegitimate children are brought into the world we must do it very humbly. No one ever completely

understands another; motives are complex; forces of social pressure, religious belief, emotional relationships within the family, private fears and longings, act in an entirely individual fashion on the individual girl according to her hereditary make up, her upbringing and the degree of her integration as a person (Wimperis, 1960, p. 97).

Explanations for these large numbers of conceptions now occurring outside marriage must take account of social and economic trends as well as the backgrounds, personalities and attitudes of the men and women concerned. No one theory will be able to account for all the circumstances leading up to the birth of a natural child; explanations have to be sought for the occurrence of extra-marital intercourse, the failure to prevent pregnancy and, now that abortion is more widely available, the continuance of the pregnancy to term. It is also mistaken to assume that unmarried mothers are a homogeneous group, or that their motives for becoming pregnant differ from those of married women (Macintyre, 1976b). Weir (1970), one of the few researchers to study a representative sample, concluded,

No particular personality type can be said to dominate. Mothers ranged from the very impulsive and carefree to the extremely careful and conscientious, from the out-going social type of individual to the lonely isolated woman; from some who are very self-critical and guilt-ridden to the rather more who are extremely critical of others and some who are social misfits. . . . The mothers came from intact homes and broken homes . . . and for every home described as unhappy there was one which claimed to be positively happy. A few mothers had but a casual acquaintance with the father of their babies; many had known him well; and for some the relationship had been a very important and deep one (p. 85).

Sexual behaviour

Undoubtedly many unplanned births occur because of the increased and widespread sexual activity amongst the young. In a study of the sexual behaviour of young people Schofield (1968) found that about 40 per cent of boys and 20 per cent of girls aged between fifteen and nineteen had some experience of sexual intercourse. Although most of these young people had some knowledge of birth control, a high proportion never took any precautions to prevent conception. The girls relied almost entirely on the boys to use a contraceptive and because of this about four-fifths of the more sexually active were at risk of becoming pregnant.

The study shows that sexual activity amongst the young was common enough to be seen as one manifestation of teenage conformity and that it is mistaken to see these sexually experienced young people as misfits or debauched. They were, however, intent on living life to the full, and sexual experience was seen by many to be a normal part of this hedonism.

This study is now somewhat out of date but it seems likely that, with increasingly permissive attitudes towards sexual'behaviour, a higher proportion of young people are now sexually active. Although contraceptives are now more easily obtainable by young unmarried people than they were in the early 1960s, the experience of other researchers and those who work with un-married mothers and single women requesting an abortion, is that a very large number of these women rarely or never use con-traception, or insist that their partner does (Lambert, 1971; Ingham and Simms, 1972).

Attitudes to sex and contraception

Many writers comment on the permissive, hedonistic and romantic attitudes, as well as the ignorance, that seem to accompany this failure to prevent unwanted pregnancies. Illsley and Gill (1968) point out that this needs to be seen in the context of an increasing acceptance of the importance and significance of sexual satisfac-tion. Given such an attitude, it seems illogical to many people to postpone this pleasure until marriage. The declining age of marriage also means that young people are in close touch with married friends who are experiencing regular and enjoyable sexual relations. For the young unmarried to be excluded from the common experience of their peers can seem unreasonable (Schofield, 1973).

The blurring of the divisions between adolescence and adulthood also contributes to the growing tendency for young people to behave in ways formerly thought to be the prerogative of adults. And yet they may reach for the symbols of adulthood without the knowledge or guidance to adopt them safely, because while society may tacitly condone this freer sexual behaviour amongst the young, it has not fully accepted as the corollary the need for efficient instruction in, and wide availability of, the safest methods of contraception. In such a context, it is inappropriate to treat the young unwed mother as a disturbed person or a moral delinquent. Williams and Hindell's study (1972), although of a relatively small sample of women, adds considerably to our knowledge about confused attitudes to contraception. One of the aims of this enquiry was to establish why it was that women, who had so little wanted to conceive that they had sought an abortion, had not used a contraceptive.

Most of the unmarried women studied were sexually in-experienced and had a highly romantic concept of relationships between the sexes which frequently did not take account of the strength of the sexual drive until it was too late. To stop to take precautions was seen as an interruption of the romantic idyll. 'It is so unnatural . . . it makes sex seem so contrived.' These attitudes persisted even when such spontaneous intercourse had given little sexual satisfaction and had resulted in unwanted pregnancy. On occasions they were part and parcel of the belief that deliberately to prepare yourself for the possibility of sexual intercourse is more a mark of immorality and promiscuity than when this occurs unplanned and by chance. Since many of the women were am-bivalent about pre-marital sex, they were not able to accept the commitment to sexual intercourse implied by getting equipped with a contraceptive. Such preparation was thought to mean that a sexual relationship might arise from lust rather than spon-taneously from a genuine loving relationship, which was seen as being the only morally acceptable one. For these girls to profess, and to believe in, their love for their sexual partners solves problems of moral ambivalence, self-respect and reputation (Rains, 1971; Luker, 1976).

Williams and Hindell's conclusions challenge popular assump-tions about a rise in the level of promiscuity.

The unmarried women in our sample were . . . striking for their lack of sexual experience and the infrequency of their sexual intercourse. The younger ones tended to have taken part in the full sexual act only once or twice, and even the most sexually experienced were having intercourse less often than the relatively inactive married women, and then only with one steady man. . . . Each current boyfriend seems to have been regarded as a possible future husband and almost all claimed to be sleeping with only one man. Almost all the respondents . . . held strongly that fidelity was essential to a sexual relationship. . . . Casual affairs were both denied and disapproved of. The unmarried women did not by any means take sex lightly; all felt that there must be some affection for the young man before being prepared to have sex with him and most also wanted to be sure of the man's affection for them. The impression was gained that, for most of the younger members of our sample at least, intercourse was agreed to fairly reluctantly and only where the relationship was felt to be stable. The pregnancy arose from beginners' ignorance and naivete. . . . Our respondents themselves tended to define promiscuity as 'sleeping around' and, in particular, sleeping with a man with whom there was no on-going bond of love. By this definition they were certainly not promiscuous, nor were they by any other definition unless the term is devalued to the point of referring to any form of pre-marital or extra-marital sex (1972, pp. 32-4).

Some women are also prevented from using contraception by the general expectation that men will play the dominant role in initiating sexual relations and that women must be pursued and wooed before agreeing to have intercourse. In such a context it can be regarded as quite inappropriate for women to anticipate their submission to masculine pressures by taking any contraceptive initiative themselves. These women run serious risks of pregnancy because of the unwillingness of men to use sheaths or withdrawal, or because of the unreliability of these methods.

It is also possible that women who can see little before them except eventual child bearing and marriage, and do not have any special commitment to work or study, feel equally little commitment to ensuring that they do not become pregnant outside marriage. Amongst this group can be found those who see pregnancy as the normal preliminary to marriage. However, the extent of such attitudes is unknown and it is highly unlikely that those to whom they apply are willing to contemplate the possibility of marriage with any man with whom they have sexual intercourse and by whom they may become pregnant.

Ignorance and knowledge

The attitudes described in the previous section reflect the education in human relationships, or more commonly the lack of this, to which most men and women have been exposed. For example, Bone (1973) found that only a third of the single women she studied said they had been taught something about intercourse and only a fifth had learnt anything about contraception. Much of the confusion about this subject reflects the generally ambivalent attitudes of society towards sexual relationships, and particularly to those of the unmarried. Although it is now recognised that the ignorance or embarrassment of many parents often makes them unsuitable as the main source of information or education about sex, there has been considerable feeling that discussion of sexual relationships should largely be confined to the home. In fact, many young people are willing only to discuss sexual matters with close friends, who may be equally ill informed. And parents' own embarrassment or ignorance means that some seem more able to cope with the crisis of an unexpected pregnancy than with the kind of unabashed discussion with their children which might help them form more circumspect relationships.

There are also some fears that discussion of sexual behaviour, and especially contraception, will encourage young people to behave in ways which would not otherwise have occurred to them. One consequence of these anxieties has been that what sexual education there is often focuses narrowly on the physiology of reproduction and is not related more widely to the whole spectrum of human relationships. The information imparted is therefore quite likely to be misunderstood, to seem irrelevant to its recipients and unrelated to meaningful notions of morality and responsibility.

Widespread ignorance, particularly among the unmarried, about sexuality and contraception is an important factor in the background to unwanted pregnancy. Many women seem to have no realistic sense of the likelihood of their becoming pregnant and thus run immense risks. For instance, infrequent or first intercourse is often thought not to result in pregnancy, and since many women have intercourse only rarely, contraception may be seen as unnecessary or not worth the effort (Williams and Hindell, 1972). Such views gain strength when, as often happens, inconsistent contraceptive practice or the use of unreliable methods do indeed appear to prevent conception. All this is compounded by a sketchy understanding of the different methods of contraception, lack of knowledge about the sources of help, and fears or actual experience of rebuff if this is sought (Pearson 1973; chapter 6).

Over and above this basic ignorance many inexperienced women appear to be taken unawares by the sexual demands of their partner and by their own sexual response. 'They told us how to do it, and why we should not do it – but nobody told us how much we'd want to do it!' (Williams and Hindell, 1972, p. 58). Some young unmarried people seem also to have no appreciation of the implications of pregnancy for them and thus have little incentive to take precautions. Adding another dimension to this problem, Bone (1973) found a considerable discrepancy between the family plans of engaged women and their contraceptive intentions. Among those who did not want to conceive as soon as they married were some who were not contemplating using contraception.

While it may be accepted that the ignorance and confusions described can help explain the sexual behaviour of the relatively unsophisticated, the unwanted pregnancies of the better educated, particularly students, are often greeted with amazement, as a symptom of apparently incomprehensible ignorance, or with disgust as a sign of obvious irresponsibility. These reactions may be far too simplistic. The well educated are just as likely as other people to be taken unawares by the strength of their sexual desires and to share the attitudes about the role of women in courtship and sexual relationships which make regular and reliable contraception problematic (McCance and Hall, 1972; Bardwick, 1973). Sophisticated and unsophisticated alike can be victims of contradictory social attitudes which extol both the value of sexual relationships and the chastity of women, while condoning the predatory or irresponsible behaviour of the fathers of natural children.

It is also possible that for some women, who feel unequal to educational and other pressures, pregnancy may appear, usually half-consciously, and certainly short-sightedly, as a kind of escape. For a girl whose education has separated her from her former peers, pregnancy may seem a confirmation to herself and to the world that she too is an ordinary woman capable of pursuing the normal pursuits of her contemporaries. Jill, described in chapter 7, is an example of such a girl.

Haphazard and careless use of contraception

That some pregnancies occur because of admitted careless or haphazard use of contraception is clear from several studies (Cartwright, 1970; Bone, 1973). The reasons often given are laziness, 'trusting to luck', a basic dislike of contraception or a particular method, fear of side effects and, more rarely, a half-acknowledged desire to become pregnant. Among the young and inexperienced this is compounded by the attitudes to sexuality and contraception already described. What may be the background to pregnancies which result from apparently deliberate carelessness?

Some women, especially those who have had a long or close relationship with their boyfriends, may admit quite openly that they wished to become pregnant, either to hasten the date of the marriage which both had planned, albeit in uncertain terms, or to bring to the fore the question of their boyfriends' commitment to them. We know that many marriages are prompted by such pregnancies. It also frequently happens that a woman quite misjudges the reaction of her boyfriend, and herself, to her pregnancy. Faced with such a crisis one or both of them may find their relationship changed and may be unwilling to proceed to a marriage which seems to have been engineered (Pearson, 1973).

Bone, finding that about a fifth of working-class girls said they were unlikely to think at all about using contraception, suggests that for some there may seem little point in avoiding conception.

> Fewer of them have the chance of a satisfying education and interesting career, and where there is no such chance their prospects will not be blighted by pregnancy. Marriage may in fact be the limit of their present ambitions and some may hope, not always unreasonably, that pregnancy will hasten the joyful day (p. 60).

'Accidental' pregnancies may also be welcomed, and half planned as a proof of fertility. Anxieties about this can be especially strong amongst those who have had an abortion, especially an illegal abortion, and who have been told that this may affect their future chances of child bearing.

Second or subsequent pregnancies which, at first sight, seem to be unplanned accidents, can at times present an attempt to replace a child 'lost' either as a result of an abortion or adoption. When pregnant for the first time these women may have received inadequate help in making up their minds about the possible courses of action before them, or they may have been subjected to various pressures not to keep the baby when they would have liked to do so. The following account of the events leading to a single girl's second pregnancy illustrates this situation well. It also shows how the birth of a child may help a woman decide on her own values and her future.

A case study: Ann, Michael and Yvonne Ann's first baby, Michael, had been placed for adoption. During her pregnancy she had been largely ostracised by her parents who were deeply ashamed of the social stigma on the family of illegitimate pregnancy. They had anyway been on bad terms with Ann for some months because of her unstable behaviour and delinquent contacts. In such a context, and bearing in mind the fact that Ann was only seventeen and quite unqualified for any job, it is perhaps unsurprising that she was advised by various doctors and welfare workers to place the child for adoption. Almost certainly this was the best decision for the baby. However, Ann did not receive much help in coping with the feelings of anger and loss which are so inextricably connected with parting with an infant. Indeed, she said she had been told that she would have to stay in an uncomfortable and somewhat primitive home for unmarried mothers until she had signed the first papers for this adoption and Michael had been taken from her. In retrospect Ann said that her anxiety to leave the home as soon as possible and to be free of the whole incident and the unpleasant events associated with it probably contributed to a hasty agreement to adoption, and certainly to her determined efforts to put the whole matter out of her mind and to suppress any feelings of sadness or regret. On leaving the home she went to London and for about a year moved from job to job and flat to flat on the assumption that a hectic life and the deliberate pursuit of pleasure were the best ways of healing her wounds.

At the end of this period Ann became pregnant by a man she knew only slightly. She never told him of the pregnancy. She also concealed it from her family and friends as long as possible, but eventually, in the eighth month of pregnancy, she was forced to turn to them and to the Social Service Department for help. At the first meetings with her social worker Ann was greatly distressed and panicky about her future. She wished she was dead and that she had got rid of the baby although apparently she had made no attempt to do this. She raged against her parents' insensitivity and rejection but wept about the shame she had brought on them. She was unwilling to discuss her more long-term future but said angrily that the hospital and the welfare could look after the baby. She never wanted to see it. She absolutely refused to talk about her earlier experiences of adoption and remained unwilling or unable to do this until several months later.

Almost immediately after the birth of her second baby, Yvonne, Ann decided, apparently out of the blue, given her previous protestations, that she wanted to keep her. She immediately and calmly proceeded to overcome all the formidable obstacles to this plan of finding suitable housing and employment, and in the process of doing this, she effected some reconciliation with her family. She continued to keep in touch with the social worker who gave her important practical help but who also found that she was increasingly being used by Ann as someone with whom she could reflect on her situation. During one of the most important conversations she gave her social worker, and perhaps herself as well, a clear insight into some of the reasons for Yvonne's conception; this baby was in some ways both a replacement for Michael and the means by which Ann was to prove herself to be a loving and responsible person.

'As you know, after all I'd gone through the first time, the last thing I wanted was to get into the same trouble again. Although I slept with several blokes I always made sure they used something. And since I didn't really want sex all that much, I wasn't too bothered about saying no. About a year after Michael was born I met Ric [Yvonne's father]. He was a nice boy although I didn't know him all that well. We only slept together a few times and I haven't seen him since. All I know is that for some reason I didn't bother to make him be careful. I remember just lying on the sofa in the dark thinking of Michael all the time and everything that had happened to us both. I suppose I wasn't too surprised to find I was pregnant although for months I tried not to think about it and pretended I wasn't. I didn't tell Ric about the baby. I think now that was because I knew he'd help me, and if he did that, then he might want to share the baby with me. I suppose it's awful to say this but I couldn't really share her with anyone yet.

'During these last few weeks that Yvonne and I have been

together I have thought about Michael most of the time. I get out the only photo I have of him and sometimes when I look at it I cry and cry. I never cried when I gave him away. Although I knew it was best for him, I wish I'd had a chance to show I loved him.

'But for Yvonne, the best thing is for her and me to stay together. I'm doing everything to make it work. I never thought I could manage so well. Even the awful bits like going to the Social Security and looking for a room I don't mind so much because I love her such a lot. It's funny isn't it, but although I feel years older and more responsible I also feel as happy as I did when I was a little girl. I don't expect I could have managed all this for Michael but it's strange and sad I had to go through all that to get like this with Yvonne.'

Unhappiness and insecurity and the wish for a child

Can we identify common elements in the backgrounds of those women for whom pregnancy can be seen as a symptom of complex personal problems or, in spite of the great cost to themselves and their families, and sometimes to the child, as purposeful behaviour? There are many accounts of the social and emotional problems of such women (Young, 1954; Rowe, 1966; Pochin, 1969). They are described as being lonely, insecure and immature with few satisfying relationships either in childhood or later life. This contributes to the dependence which makes it difficult for many to develop as individuals in their own right, and which leaves them tied to their parents despite the unhappiness surrounding these relationships. As a consequence many become vulnerable to the suggestion or fantasy that a boyfriend and a sexual relationship will remove their loneliness, even when such liaisons seem likely to be transitory or unsatisfying. Those who are drawn to these kinds of relationships are unlikely to take contraceptive precautions.

There are also women for whom the pregnancy and child appear to be far more important than the relationship with the father. In these cases a girl's pregnancy can sometimes be seen, in part, as an assertion of her independence, as giving her her own identity. Alternatively, a girl may be hoping that with her baby she will find the love that has so far eluded her. For all these women there is the expectation, although sometimes only dimly perceived, that pregnancy and a child will bring release from family tensions and personal unhappiness; and this seems to promote an almost blind disregard of the problems so closely associated with the birth and care of an illegitimate child.

The context of these explanations

Until recently it was common for social workers to explain the pregnancies of most, if not all, single unsupported women in such terms. Most of the books and research studies written twenty or thirty years ago, which have been extremely influential in some professional circles, emphasise the high degree of social and personal pathology in the backgrounds of unmarried mothers. In many of these there is a striking lack of interest in such contributory factors as the problems associated with the use of contraception.

This somewhat narrow focus has to be understood in its social context. When there are relatively strong pressures on young women not to have pre-marital sexual relations it is likely that those who fail to conform will be seen as unusual, and various explanations will be sought for their unconventional behaviour. To focus on the motivations of single girls to have babies represents an attempt, most important and much needed, to challenge the sometimes sentimental or ill-informed stereotypes of unmarried mothers as either the innocent victims of predatory men or as over-sexed women whose uncontrollable urges make them careless and undiscriminating in their sexual relations. Since such explanations frequently fail to fit the facts, they tend to result in help being offered which is either too limited or quite inappropriate.

Another reason for the widespread currency among social workers of the view of unmarried mothers as disturbed people is the fact that they, as well as many researchers, are more likely to be brought into contact with women who seek help because their own problems make it impossible for them to cope with their pregnancy and child unaided.

It may also be that the need for social workers to make the best of things, to come to terms with the inevitable and to salvage something of value from what may seem at first sight a disastrous situation, puts pressure on them to regard all behaviour as having purpose and meaning. To see a perfect baby as truly unwanted challenges deeply held beliefs and emotions and encourages a will to believe that the child *must* be wanted, even though the reasons may be obscure, confused or irrational.

Understandable and, in certain respects, laudable though this type of explanation may be, it has to be regarded as inadequate by itself. A change in sexual morals such as has occurred in the last twenty years or so clearly challenges explanations which focus narrowly on women's wish or need for a child, and most workers are now aware of the need to adopt a more sophisticated approach in attempts to understand the background to illegitimacy. As Bernstein (1966) remarks, it should be obvious that a girl may become an unmarried mother because she has pre-existing problems, or she may have problems because she is an unmarried mother. If we adopt a frame of reference which assumes that illegitimacy is invariably a symptom of underlying emotional problems, we will be on the alert for such difficulties; we are likely to convince ourselves that we have found them; and we may proceed to interpret all the behaviour of an unmarried mother in such terms (Macintyre, 1976a). Rowe (1966), however, draws attention to a group of pregnant girls who are unmarried but largely free from emotional disturbance, and the evidence of other researchers shows that only a minority, perhaps less than a quarter, of unmarried mothers can be identified as having serious emotional or family problems (Vincent, 1961; Yelloly, 1964). It is possible that the more frequent occurrence of pre-marital sexual relations in the last ten years means that this proportion is now lower.

These criticisms of explanations which rely exclusively on motivation and personal pathology warn us against their in-discriminate application. This should not obscure the fact that such explanations can be extremely useful in attempting to un-derstand the pregnancies of women who seem very ambivalent about what course of action they should take; of those who are at a loss to explain how they became pregnant; of the older, educated or sophisticated women whose pregnancies would seem, at first sight, to be a social and personal disaster which apparently they could have avoided; of some of those who repeatedly con-ceive outside marriage; and of the girls who seem caught in a web of unhappy family relationships. In some circumstances these explanations throw light on behaviour that is apparently meaningless, self-centred and self-damaging, and can alert workers to the importance of designing help which takes account of the complex needs and emotions contributing to such behaviour.

Emotional deprivation and relationships with parents

Mothers and daughters

It is not uncommon for single pregnant women to have poor relationships with their mothers, and, less frequently, with their fathers. Some of these women seem to have been more or less rejected early in life, with many of the most deprived spending their childhood in institutions or homes. The hunger for affection and their emotional immaturity makes them undiscriminating in the choice of partners and unable to share in a loving and lasting relationship. It sometimes seems as if these girls' choice of such friends as married men with families, or young boys who are probably unwilling or unable to maintain a lasting liaison with them, indicates that it is a baby rather than an adult relationship which is sought as a consolation and a focus of love and affection. Not all women will be explicit about their hopes and fantasies of their future, although they may behave in ways which ensure that their pregnancy will go to term. While there are many reasons for concealing a pregnancy, long delays in asking for help, which might include the suggestion that a pregnancy should be terminated, may indicate that a woman wishes to keep the child.

Other women, perhaps the more disturbed, do not seem able to visualise the child as a distinct individual, with his or her own needs and personality. Although such women appear to possess a very strong desire to have a baby, often at great cost to themselves, they seem to have little concern for its future. The baby comes to be a symbol of a girl's long unrecognised need to be seen as a woman; or it may be a weapon in a complicated battle with parents.

These girls' sexual partners are often described in the haziest fashion; neither their Christian nor surname may be known and the relationships appear fleeting and unimportant. Such men appear only to be biological necessities, to be discarded once they have fulfilled their function of impregnating the woman. In such circumstances contraception seems utterly remote from women's minds, and queries about it will either be ignored or greeted with blank amazement.

Emotional deprivation can take many forms, but it is common to find the lives of these disturbed and unhappy women dominated by their own parents, and especially by their mothers. Within these families relationships are often extremely complicated, and underlying superficial pronouncements of solidarity and affection are possessiveness, envy and jealousy, fear and dislike. For some girls the crisis of pregnancy provides a means of extricating themselves from such a situation; others are less successful and they and their children remain caught in a tangle of family pathology. Young described these girls as

> usually very passive, lacking in the capacity to make conscious decisions and unable to use more than a small fraction of their abilities. Colourless in personality, they are almost completely prisoners of their own prohibitions, unable to establish more than the most superficial relationships with anyone except on a dependent, small child-to-mother basis. . . . [They] tend to be more or less passive, fearful of decisive action, incapable of spontaneous self-expression, over-absorbed in their own fears, conflicts and fantasies. All of them to some degree feel that they have no right to any life, will or wishes of their own . . . (1954, p. 51).

This passivity is apparent in some girls' explanations of the relationship which resulted in their pregnancy. They deny, often quite absurdly, taking any part in initiating or continuing it and tell stories of rape, amnesia, or 'knock-out drops'. These accounts may also be prompted by very genuine fears of a mother's hostile reactions to her daughter's disgraceful and uncharacteristic behaviour and implicit assertion of her femininity. Many mothers wish to return as soon as possible to the situation in which their daughters present no threat to them. They are anxious to dispose of the baby, either through adoption or abortion, and try to organise their daughters' lives completely, with the latter's apparently total acquiescence in this state of affairs.

Paradoxically, in spite of these mothers' rage and distress, and initial assertion that they will have nothing whatever to do with the baby, it is not at all unusual for them to take over the child, and proceed to care for him or her with exclusive and smothering affection. And those girls who vowed they could never tell their mothers about their pregnancies because 'the shock would kill her', eventually seem to anticipate this apparently quite unexpected reaction and appear unsurprised by the volte-face. Some relinquish their babies into their mothers' hands with relief, almost with a sense of accomplishment, as if this had been the ultimate aim of their pregnancy. The baby becomes a substitute for the daughter who is now freed to live a more independent life. Others, perhaps the more mature and stable, for whom the pregnancy and the baby are insufficient assertions of their independence, resist all attempts to limit their own maternal responsibilities. They seek a life outside the confines of their family and the loving relationship they have not found with their parents; this often seems more possible with a small child than it does with a man.

Fathers and daughters

It is the fathers of some unmarried mothers who seem to be the chief source of their unhappiness. They appear to their daughters as cruel, rejecting or tyrannical, sometimes ill-treating their wives and children who may be drawn together for self-protection and in shared dislike of this dominant member of the household. Not surprisingly, many girls who live in the shadow of such distorted relationships develop a contempt for the opposite sex; their memories of their fathers as selfish or sadistic are projected quite indiscriminately onto all males. For some this means a series of masochistic relationships which confirm their image of themselves as unworthy and unlovable. If they become pregnant or make any demands of their partners, they are almost certain to be deserted.

There are also some girls whose hatred for their father leads them to punish men by using a pregnancy or a baby to damage a former lover. Such a girl may publicise the fact of his paternity so as to wreck his home life or employment, even when she has engineered the pregnancy, does not wish to marry the man and has been offered support for herself and her child. Girls with this background are among the most disturbed of unmarried mothers. They frequently have few strong feelings for their babies but a determination to use them for as long as possible as weapons in their own private battles with men.

Only a minority of unmarried mothers have experienced these pathological relationships. Much more common are those women whose backgrounds are not nearly so disturbed but whose unhappiness or insecurity may be associated with pregnancy outside marriage. Some of these women may have committed themselves to success in work or education to the exclusion of deep personal relationships; for them a pregnancy may represent a crossroads in their life, where they must reflect on their past and future priorities. An older woman may willingly have devoted herself to the care of her parents but regret the bleakness of her emotional life. Despite acute social embarrassment, for her a child may seem a protection against loneliness. Other women may, for a variety of reasons, find it difficult to express emotion and to make satisfying relationships. For them a baby may act as a catalyst, the focus of deep feelings and a bridge to other relationships. Rosamund in Margaret Drabble's novel, *The Millstone*, is a single girl who begins to face and solve some of her personal problems when she becomes a mother.

> At times I had a vague complicated sense that this pregnancy had been sent to me in order to reveal to me a scheme of things totally different from the scheme which I inhabited ... it was as though too long I had been living in one way, on one plane and the way I had ignored had been forced thus abruptly and violently to assert itself. . . . I am sure that my discoveries were common discoveries. . . . The only curious feature in my case is that the facts I now discovered were precisely the same facts that my admirable parents had always so firmly presented to our childish eyes: facts of inequality, of limitation, of separation, of the impossible, heart-breaking, uneven hardship of the human lot. I had always felt for others in theory and pitied the blows of fate and circumstances under which they suffered; but now, myself no longer free, myself suffering, I may say that I felt it in my heart ... I saw that from now on I ... was going to have to ask for help, and from strangers too: I who could not even ask for love or friendship ... Gradually I began to realise that she [her baby] liked me, and that unless I took great pains to alienate her she would go on liking me, for a couple of years at least. It was very pleasant to receive such uncritical love because it left me free to bestow love. . . . Indeed, it must have been in expectation of this love that I had insisted upon having her, or rather refrained from not having her: something in me had clearly known before I did that there would be compensations (pp. 67-8, 72, 115).

Pregnancy in young girls

> Unhappiness and emotional deprivation in the family may lead
> the girl to develop a morbid craving to be wanted, to be loved
> and to have someone or something to love. Both a boyfriend
> and a baby may be sought as compensation and as a
> reassurance that to be unwanted and a failure are not
> necessary conditions of life (Lane Report, 1974, para. 236).

In the Western world pregnancy in school-age girls has long been
regarded as a matter of serious concern, as a symptom of acute
personal and social pathology. These views have been formed
largely by the various professional workers closely concerned with
the problems of school-aged mothers. There has been no thorough
research into the backgrounds of these girls although recent
evidence, from small studies, tends to confirm the impression that
pregnancy in schoolgirls is often associated with a multiplicity of
personal and social problems, very little sex education and the
inability of the girl and her parents to communicate with each
other (Russell, 1970; Horobin *et al.*, 1973). Some of these girls,
whose craving for love has not been fulfilled at home, seek this
from their boyfriends, and subsequently from their babies
(Gough, 1964 and 1966).

> They hoped to satisfy their wish to feel needed, loved and
> good, not only in the arms of their boyfriends, but also through
> their babies' need and love of them, through the compassion
> and interest which they hoped their new motherhood would
> arouse and through the reassurance that they would get from
> producing a healthy and good baby (Gough, 1966, p. 6).

These expectations may sometimes be realised. There is some
evidence that young pregnant girls' relationships with their
boyfriends, who are usually about two or three years older, have
often been established for several months or even a year or two
before a child has been conceived. Although the immaturity of the
partners means that they would be unwise to marry, a fact they
themselves frequently point out, their friendships are often a
source of mutual consolation and satisfaction. When the pregnancy is discovered these relationships tend to be disrupted, often
inappropriately, by parental pressures. When the bonds are strong

enough to survive these crises some workers now believe that it can be helpful for both the young people, with support and guidance, to continue their relationship (Smith, 1966).

We cannot be so sanguine about the prospects of school-age motherhood as a solution to personal problems. Although many young girls care well for their infants physically and form attachments to them, very few are able to provide adequate homes, especially if they are unsupported by their own families. They are also usually too immature to meet the demands of toddlers and older children. Indeed, it would be quite wrong to thrust such responsibilities on them.

Awareness of these problems has led workers to favour plans which relieve the very young mother of the long-term care of her child, preferably through adoption. This arrangement, although often ideal for the infant, can be fraught with problems for the mother and her family. Apart from social embarrassment, by no means a trivial problem to many people, a pregnancy can seriously disrupt a girl's education. It usually means as well as acute personal distress, the making of hard decisions and tension at home. Parting from a baby who is to be adopted and the subsequent feelings of loss and guilt must always be painful. For very young mothers with disturbed backgrounds and few family supports this suffering is particularly acute. They have little hope of alternative consolations or loving care.

Given all these difficulties it is not surprising that almost three-quarters (in 1974 70 per cent) of pregnant schoolgirls now have abortions. This may provide the best, although often only a partial, solution to a difficult problem. Although it may prevent the deterioration of serious social and personal difficulties, it cannot remove them. Too speedy or automatic decisions to terminate the pregnancies of young girls can mean ignoring these problems, with the risk that they will precipitate further pregnancies, especially if a girl never really wanted an abortion but was unable to resist the various pressures persuading her that this was the right course of action (Horobin et al., 1973).

Increasing sexual experimentation among the young and the raising of the school-leaving age mean that school-age pregnancy will probably become more commonplace, and not simply the product of grossly disturbed families. Nevertheless, a young girl's pregnancy will inevitably bring all kinds of social and emotional problems. Social attitudes towards the sexual activity of young people, especially when this is confirmed by pregnancy, their educational needs, the difficulties of making decisions about their own future, and most painfully, that of their child, plus the shock and anxieties of their parents mean that even the most stable young people and their families are likely, temporarily at least, to be overwhelmed.

Bearing in mind all these dilemmas the Lane Committee recommended that young pregnant girls and their families should receive special attention and care. They also warned against exaggerating the extent of this problem, serious though it must be for each individual. Pregnancies and abortions to girls under sixteen only make up a tiny proportion (just over 2 per cent) of all extra-marital pregnancies. In 1974 there were over 1,400 births to girls under sixteen; there were also more than 3,000 abortions in the same age group. This means that out of every 1,000 young girls at risk only two actually became pregnant.

Illegitimacy and decisions about abortion

In 1973 the pregnancies of rather more than half the single women under twenty years of age were terminated. Among those who had their babies will be some who had asked for, but been refused, an abortion. Their circumstances may not be so different from those of women whose pregnancies have been terminated, and their desire for an abortion may have been as great. The fact that their pregnancies went to term is a reflection of doctors' differing interpretations of the Abortion Act and variations in the availability of abortion (chapter 6). Women considering an abortion are more or less likely to obtain this depending on where they live, and if this is an area where abortion is not readily available within the National Health Service, on whether they can afford private treatment. Although it is important to remember that the ease with which a woman is put off pursuing a request for abortion may reflect how determined she is not to have a baby, the obstacles confronting some women should not be underestimated (Lafitte, 1975). Not the least of these are idiosyncratic views about the pregnancies of single women. The sexual behaviour of the unmarried can provoke punitive attitudes and refusals to terminate the pregnancies of those regarded as immoral or irresponsible. Decisions about abortion may also be made on the basis of extremely dubious understanding of the implications of unmarried motherhood for different social groups which may exclude or distort the assessment of any individual woman's particular situation (Horobin *et al.*, 1973).

To an extent, therefore, the births of some natural children may be regarded as chance events, the results of the medical treatment the mother has been able to obtain. This fact should be borne in mind by those who are inclined to see the birth of a natural child largely as a symptom of the mother's serious social and emotional problems and as her attempt to solve these.

Some areas of ignorance

The fathers of natural children

If what is known about sexual behaviour and family dynamics, about contraception and medical practice, underlines the complexities in understanding the background to illegitimacy, these are compounded by ignorance in several important areas. First and foremost, attempting to explain single women's sexual behaviour and attitudes to motherhood is hazardous when so little is known about their partners. Largely because pregnancy and the care of a child do not impinge directly, or at all, on the father's life, his role in fathering the child and his subsequent responsibility for his offspring have received little attention; Vincent (1961) estimates that twenty-five times more research has been conducted into the behaviour and backgrounds of unmarried mothers than into those of unmarried fathers. To some extent this lack of interest reflects traditional attitudes towards sexual behaviour of men and their responsibility for their children. It has been considered more or less normal, and indeed necessary, for men to have a wider range of sexual relationships than would be generally permissible for women. Freedom to experiment with sexuality is condoned even though it results in the conception of large numbers of unwanted children. This complacency means that little or no attention has been paid to such questions as why greater sexual freedom should be thought necessary for men, what kind of women are chosen as partners for casual or experimental affairs, why men do not use contraception, whether they actually wish to father children, and how they react to the knowledge that their partner has conceived a child.

It is widely assumed that most men wish to escape the financial and other commitments which flow from admitting they have fathered a natural child. They therefore tend to be viewed with hostile suspicion, or to be totally ignored. But excluding men from decisions about their children's future, treating their irresponsibilities with indulgence, or hounding them to pay what can sometimes seem a fine for a sexual transgression, regardless of the circumstances of a particular situation, are hardly conducive to responsible and considerate behaviour towards the girl and the baby. In fact, the experience of many workers is that men frequently wish to be involved in planning for their child, and the majority will admit paternity and offer some financial or other practical help if they can discuss the situation fully, and from their own point of view (Smith, 1966; Pochin, 1969).

Such a conclusion is hardly surprising, unless it is believed that men in general care little for their sexual partners and have no feelings for their unintended offspring. Numerous studies show that many of the relationships which have resulted in an unwanted pregnancy are long lasting and deeply important to the couple. And it is hardly sensible to imagine that the reactions of one half of the population towards parenthood are quite unlike those of the other. If allowed the opportunity, unmarried fathers can show the deepest concern for their children, and in spite of the prejudices against them, at least a few would like to take the major responsibility for their care (Barber, 1975).

There is little reliable information about the background to unmarried fatherhood. Young (1954) suggests that if more attempt was made to see these fathers as troubled people, rather than as sources of cash or ruthless seducers to be pilloried, they would be found to have problems and personalities which complement those of their partners. When pregnancy is associated with the kind of unhappy and neurotic situations described earlier in this chapter, it is certainly possible that the men and women concerned will have selected each other because of the similarity of their backgrounds and needs (Smith, 1966).

What influences the plans of single parents?

Little is known about the factors which influence the intentions of single men and women concerning the children they have conceived. What circumstances prompt a request for an abortion? How much general knowledge is there about its availability and consequences; or about the problems of caring for a child as a single parent; or about the assistance available to people in this situation? What makes it more possible for some women than others to envisage placing their infants for adoption, and to stand by this decision?

In the absence of hard information, answers to these questions tend to be riddled with prejudice. For example, although it is assumed that relatively liberal legal abortion practices will quickly become well known, thus influencing to some extent the choices women make about their unwanted pregnancies, Horobin et al. (1973) found that in Aberdeen few women had a sophisticated knowledge about the availability of abortion in their home area, in spite of the liberal policy of the local consultants during the previous ten years. By contrast, it is often asserted that single women seem to think that abortion is always available, just for the asking, the inference being that they had few anxieties about unwanted pregnancies. Pearson (1973) has produced some evidence which contradicts this somewhat cold-blooded view. In his study of the social and psychological aspects of extra-marital first conceptions he found that the majority of women saw abortion as a last resort; most of those having an abortion would have preferred marriage and motherhood, although for many these were not real possibilities because of uncertain or unhappy relationships with the child's father. Those who opted for abortion rather than continuing the pregnancy were more likely to have accepted it. This decision was also closely associated with concern about the stigma of having a natural child and the distress this would cause close relatives.

Like several other researchers Pearson found that offering the child for adoption was generally the least favoured of the possible alternatives, with many women forcibly expressing aversion to this. The origins of this unpopularity are not clear. It is certainly possible that the greater availability of abortion has had some influence, although the number of children being offered for adoption was declining before the Abortion Act was passed (Triseliotis, 1971). We also do not know whether those factors associated with a decision to place a child for adoption, which were studied by Yelloly (1965), still apply now that abortion is more readily available. Do mothers whose social circumstances or parents' negative attitudes would formerly have predisposed them to adoption, now opt for abortion? Is it still true, as Yelloly and other workers suggest, that the more unstable and disturbed mothers are also more likely to keep their children? Are those women who decide to keep their natural children aware of the hardships and risks this is likely to entail? And if they are what makes them decide that there is more to be gained than lost by facing these?

These gaps in our knowledge can begin to be filled by the observations of individual workers. Their conclusions, if founded on a sensitive understanding of men's and women's reactions to the dilemmas of an unwanted pregnancy, may well challenge prejudiced or outdated assumptions.

The future of natural children

They were beset by a multiplicity of unfavourable circumstances which not only gave them a relatively poorer start in life but which continued to build up into a complex web of cumulative and interacting disadvantages and deprivations. Thus at the present time, to be born illegitimate is still to be born disadvantaged (Crellin et al., 1971, p. 112).

While there is still much we do not know about the background to illegitimacy, there have been many studies of natural children. Although the difficulties they face are by no means unique, and in particular may be shared by the children of other single-parent families, natural children are especially vulnerable to a series of economic and emotional deprivations from their earliest babyhood.

The clearest evidence for this comes from the National Child Development Study, carried out by the National Children's Bureau, which is one of the most thorough studies ever conducted of the comparative development of children. Part of this research compared the physical, educational and emotional development of legitimate and natural children. Comparisons were also made between natural children cared for by their mothers, those who were brought up by adoptive parents and those living with grandparents or in care. In almost all respects, by the age of seven, the natural children who remained with their mothers fared significantly worse than legitimate children; by contrast the natural children who had been adopted did better than both groups. These findings were largely independent of other variables, such as social class (Crellin, 1971). Reports of the subsequent development of these children have yet to be published.

Partly because of their mothers' youth, and because ante-natal care was often sought relatively late in pregnancy, the death and prematurity rates for natural children were, in 1958, some 60 per cent greater than those of the legitimate babies; twice as many natural babies were also found to have a low birth weight (less than 2,500 grams). These problems were particularly severe for the children of unsupported single mothers who were the most likely during pregnancy to suffer from social and emotional stress. At the age of seven the natural unadopted children lived in far less favourable circumstances than did their peers. The homes of one in seven had no father-figure compared with only 2 per cent of those of other children. A third lived in homes which lacked some of the most basic amenities, such as hot water or an inside lavatory. Only 17 per cent of the legitimate and 5 per cent of the adopted children lived in such circumstances. Nearly a quarter of the natural children lived in overcrowded conditions, and over 40 per cent of the unsupported mothers of natural children suffered from financial hardship.

The majority of the mothers of natural children went out to work, both to achieve a higher standard of living than that possible on social security, and to relieve the monotony and loneliness of single parenthood. However, the general problems women experience in finding reasonably paid, congenial employment, problems which are exacerbated when they have young children, resulted in a marked degree of downward social mobility for these families. Their children were also likely to experience some form of substitute day care. While this in itself need not be detrimental, the shortage and expense of high standard day care meant that many natural children were exposed to varying degrees of emotional and intellectual deprivation. That all these problems persist is clear from the researches of the Finer Committee (1974).

In spite of the fact that many of the natural children were living in two-parent families (though not usually with both their own parents), one in nine, compared with one in fifty of the whole sample, had come into care, usually before five years of age and usually more than once.

It is to the credit of the mothers of the natural children that these unfavourable circumstances did not appear to affect their physical development, which was found to be similar to that of the other children. But in other aspects of measurable ability and attainment, such as reading ability, general knowledge and creative development, no matter what their social background, the natural children did far less well than the legitimate and the adopted. In their general behaviour and adjustment the natural children also showed evidence of greater difficulties than the other two groups. Surprisingly, this poor performance was as typical of natural children whose mothers had married, or who were cohabiting – the vast majority in the study – as it was of those living only with their mothers.

Lacking proper control groups and long-term follow-up, earlier studies of natural children tended to assume that although they were vulnerable to all kinds of social and emotional hazards while their mothers remained single, these problems would largely disappear if their mothers married or were regularly supported by a man. Why does this apparently common-sense conclusion appear, from Crellin's findings, to be false?

Part of the answer to this question may lie in these children's experience of fathering. This subject has been almost entirely neglected, and we can, therefore, only draw inferences from the little research there is on the effects of paternal deprivation on children living with two parents. Andry (1971) found that delinquent boys were far more likely than non-delinquents to have poor relationships with their fathers. He reports that, compared with the control groups, delinquent boys received less strong and open affection from their parents, and especially from their fathers. There was poor communication and limited contacts between these fathers and their sons, and they lived in homes dominated by tension, to which their fathers contributed a considerable share. Both the boys and their parents were aware of these inadequacies.

These conclusions about the importance of a father's influence on his children may well be relevant to the many families where a natural child is cared for by his mother and official or unofficial stepfather. While these fathers are often able to accept, and love as their own, someone else's child, there are many potential problems in such a relationship for all the members of the family (Maddox, 1975). It is therefore likely that some of these children will be deprived of paternal affection and interest.

It is also possible that, in some families at least, the problems of single mothers, which must inevitably affect their offspring, are too great simply to be removed by marriage. Weir (1970) studied the factors influencing a mother's decision about the future of her child. Her enquiry took account of many earlier studies which showed mothers and their natural children to be beset by numerous social and emotional problems. The poverty and environmental stress of these single-parent families resulted in large numbers of children being taken into care. Children cared for by relatives or by foster parents were also likely to face various emotional problems (Wimperis, 1960).

Weir's findings, to some extent, confirmed these depressing conclusions. She found, as Vincent had done in America, that although there were some differences between the age groups, in general, in the 1960s, the mothers who kept their babies were more likely to belong to the lower socio-economic groups and to have disturbed family backgrounds than those girls who gave up their children for adoption. Because these women tended to move away from their parents, they also lacked financial and emotional support they might have been able to give. Weir concludes that 'To these women, their babies represent the most important primary relationship they have' (p. 66). Sadly, because of a combination of their own family circumstances and the absence of adequate welfare services, their efforts to meet their own emotional needs in this way rendered themselves and their children extremely vulnerable.

In addition, some single mothers may be more than usually at risk of hasty or ill-considered marriage. The pressures to marry, to ease financial hardships, and to escape the daunting prospect of coping unaided with the numerous everyday crises of family life, are very great. Even an uncertain relationship may seem to hold the promise of protection and support. Contrary to expectations, Crellin found that the small minority of children whose mothers remained unsupported fared relatively well. Perhaps they bear witness to the enterprise and efforts of a particularly able and resilient group of women, who prefer managing on their own to embarking on hazardous relationships.

All these problems are exacerbated by the natural child's uncertain legal status. The father of a natural child is only bound to support him after a legally enforceable order (usually an affiliation order) has been made. A number of complicated regulations surround the making of these orders. The mother also has to take the initiative herself, in a public court, both to obtain an order and to ask for it to be enforced if a father does not maintain his contributions. After all these efforts the maximum sum that can be awarded is small. All this means that only a minority of mothers are assured of regular financial help from the fathers of their children, and led Wimperis (1960) to the depressing conclusion that only 'Twelve per cent of fathers pay less than two thirds of the sum fixed. Which is half the sum that might be fixed. And less than a quarter maintain payment' (p. 143). Fourteen years later the Finer Committee were equally unimpressed by the potential of affiliation orders as a source of income for unmarried mothers.

Except for a child adopted by his relatives or natural parents, or when his mother marries, by her and her husband, natural children have only one relative legally responsible for them – their mother. They do not count in law as a member of either fathers' or mothers' families. There are no provisions in Britain, as there are in Scandinavian countries, for the State to assume any special responsibility for the protection and care of natural children. Apart from the obvious financial insecurity inherent in this situation, natural children still suffer from the stigma of illegitimacy.

It is essential to remember that it is by no means inevitable that any individual natural child will experience the problems described so far. Through their parents' efforts, or the support of other relatives or friends, or because of their own personalities and gifts, many overcome all the obstacles to a fulfilling and successful life. Adversity can bring forth extraordinary courage (Parker, 1972). Nevertheless, it is clear that, as a group, natural children are particularly vulnerable. They should, therefore, receive priority treatment from the social services. The inadequacies of this help is the theme of the next section.

Social services and the unsupported mother

There ... [are] ... girls and women who in easier
circumstances might have made good mothers, but because of
their low earning power and housing difficulties and the need
to be out most of the day earning their living, could not be
the good mothers they longed to be (Wimperis 1960, p. 118).

There is little doubt that social stigma continues to be
attached to illegitimacy, as does the view that women finding

themselves in this position must expect to suffer the consequences of their action. In addition, single mothers share the economic and emotional hardships experienced by all groups of unsupported mothers (Wimperis, 1960; Wynn, 1964; Marsden, 1969; Holman, 1970). But whereas widows and deserted wives are likely to be given sympathy and support by relatives and friends, the unmarried mother often has to cope without either (Crellin, 1971, p. 114).

In the last fifteen years there have been several studies of un-supported women and their children. Their conclusions make sober reading, particularly since these families' circumstances have improved little during this period. Moreover, the number of lone women with dependent children receiving supplementary benefit increased more than four times between 1960 and 1975 (Finer Report, 1974, vol. 1, part 5).

Most unsupported mothers face financial hardships and all of them have to contend with complex social and emotional problems. Wimperis (1960), in her study of unmarried mothers, found that those women who did not go out to work faced living on a bare subsistence income, often in extreme loneliness. The mothers who worked often had to take poorly paid jobs, where the conditions of employment roughly approximated to the availability of child-minding services. Only a minority were able to find substitute care for their children which they could afford, and this was frequently of a low standard, involving frequent moves for the child. All mothers had acute difficulties in finding accommodation and this was often totally inadequate for their most basic needs. In contradiction to widespread assumptions that natural children can be successfully incorporated into their grandparents' home, with their mothers going out to work and taking only partial responsibility for them, Wimperis found many mothers unhappy with this solution. There were problems of differing expectations of behaviour and discipline, rivalry for the child's affection and confusion about identity and parental rela-tionships.

Ten years later Holman (1970) found all these problems to be continuing, a particularly depressing conclusion in view of the fact that his study probably included a disproportionate number of educated and capable women. These attainments did not protect them from poverty and numerous other hardships. Nearly a third had incomes below the minimum set by the Supplementary Benefits Commission, usually because those who preferred to work than to live on social security could only command extremely low wages. Most of the other mothers had barely adequate incomes. The poorest women were the unmarried with young babies.

Few mothers could find the type of substitute care they most wanted for their children, usually a place in a nursery or a nursery school. As a consequence, some mothers decided against going out to work in spite of the social isolation and feelings of inadequacy and dependence this involved. Many others were 'forced to use daily minders, or occasionally to have their children privately fostered and there were criticisms of this kind of care (Holman, 1973; Jackson, 1976).

Again, despite its apparent advantages, care of children by relatives proved unpopular. As well as the difficulties described by Wimperis, many mothers found intolerable the strain of being grateful to their parents, while disagreeing with their methods of child care. They also resented, although they sometimes understood, their parents' restrictions on their use of free time; many were not expected to go out lest 'they should get into trouble again'. And they were anxious that as their children grew beyond the baby stage, their grandparents would be less able or less willing to care for them.

Although all lone mothers have similar responsibilities, a woman's marital status can have a significant influence on her income. There are many anomalies in the social security system which work against the interests of certain groups of unsupported mothers, especially the unmarried (Wynn, 1964; Marsden, 1969; Finer Report, 1974). To rectify these the Finer Committee proposed a Guaranteed Maintenance Allowance payable to all lone parents, whatever their marital status. These proposals have been turned down by the Government partly, it is said, because of their cost. There may also be some opposition to social security allowances which both acknowledge and support, without discrimination, family units which do not accord with ordinary conventions. However, until such allowances are forthcoming, a child's fatherlessness, or motherlessness, will not be the main or only determinant of the family's welfare benefits.

A woman's marital status may also influence the attitudes of officials who make decisions about social security payments (Marsden, 1969; Stevenson, 1972). While the plight of widows draws sympathy and understanding, unmarried mothers or separated women challenge conventional morality. This can complicate relationships between the officials and some unsupported mothers, who may be sensitive to any hint of criticism, and whose perceptions of the workings of the social security system are often

> shaped by the emotional turmoil of their broken relationships, by their anxious hopes and painful needs, their preconceptions about the nature of 'public' assistance, their pride and their feelings about how the rest of the population looked at them (Marsden, 1969, pp. 177-8).

In such a situation it is not surprising that some confused and apparently unfair decisions about social security are made, leaving some women resentful of their dependence on public assistance and doubtful about their rights.

The considerable physical and emotional struggles involved in maintaining even a low standard of living are made infinitely harder to bear by women's anxiety that their children should not suffer, either absolutely, or by comparison with their peers. In an affluent society where treats and small luxuries are commonplace it is inevitable that mothers will be badgered to provide these extras, and that they and their children should feel acutely the shame of obvious poverty. Children make their own comparisons. They compete to be the same, and even when, at considerable personal cost, their mothers provide a standard of living adequate for their health and general development, it is painful, in the midst of affluence, to be unable to provide the special clothes and food, the outings and the pocket money which are the normal part of other children's lives.

Some women, aware of all these difficulties and feeling either inadequate to cope with them, or unwilling to risk their children's happiness, decide to place their babies for adoption. This is not a popular solution. There is the dread of the pain of separation and the fear that, when it comes to the point, a mother will be unable to part with her baby. To some women it seems more immoral to give birth to a child they cannot support themselves, than to have their pregnancies terminated. Horobin et al. (1973) found that over 60 per cent of the women they studied whose babies were adopted had some regrets about these arrangements; and half of those who were glad about the adoption severely regretted having continued with their pregnancies. However, Triseliotis's study of a similar group of mothers came to rather different conclusions (1971).

The choices before a single pregnant woman are therefore unenviable. Both abortion and adoption involve irrevocable and often painful decisions. Unpleasant though these options may be women often feel driven to them as preferable alternatives to the hazards and responsibilities of bringing up a child alone. To fail in this enterprise may have dire consequences. And failure may have little to do with a woman's capabilities, but be the product of a welfare system and social environment unequal to a mother's aspirations (Mandell, 1973; Holman, 1975; Cheetham, 1976).

Reception into care

Perhaps some of the mothers and children who suffer most are those who live in the shadow of sporadic or protracted separation, a fate which is obviously more common when there are no relatives to help out in family crisis. Any separation is distressing for a child but if this only lasts a short time the consequences are unlikely to be severe or long lasting (Heinicke and Westheimer, 1966; Rutter, 1972). More serious are those separations which were intended to be temporary but which have become protracted, either because the mother's circumstances make it impossible for the child to return to her, or because emotional difficulties between the mother and child, often a direct consequence of separation, make reunions unsuccessful. Many of the mothers who face the worst difficulties are those whose babies are placed in temporary foster care while they make plans for their future. Some of these women may have intended their babies to be adopted but cannot bring themselves to give their final consent. Others may have been overwhelmed by the practical and emotional problems of caring unsupported for their children, difficulties which they may not fully have faced while pregnant. The longer a child remains in supposedly temporary foster care the harder it becomes for a woman to make a decision about his or her long-term future. While this uncertainty persists the child is also more likely to be transferred from foster to residential care.

The consequences of long-term institutional care have been much studied. They vary according to the age of the child at reception into care, the type of institution and the contact that can be continued with the family. Although it would be wrong to draw simple conclusions about an extremely complex subject there is reasonable evidence that life in such surroundings increases the likelihood of behaviour problems, often means the absence of close or continuous relationships, and can lead to problems of identity for the child (Dinnage and Pringle, 1967). Even if these problems are avoided life in the institution, with constantly changing staff, must almost inevitably be a bleak experience (Sinclair, 1956; Norman, 1969; Timms, 1973). To avoid the recognised hazards of residential care it is generally agreed that most children should be cared for within a family, and that if this cannot be their own, then they should live in an adoptive or foster home which will provide a reasonable degree of intimacy and permanency. How successful are the social services in achieving this aim?

For a number of reasons the answer to this question cannot be optimistic. Many children remain in care primarily because their parents lack the material resources to provide an adequate home. The worst problem, and the most difficult for the individual and the social services to solve, is shortage of accommodation. Children also remain for long periods in residential care because it is feared that a foster home placement would be unfair to the foster parents and the child if the natural mother decides, perhaps somewhat randomly, to remove him or her from care. This she has been legally entitled to do if her child was received into care on a voluntary basis. The 1975 Children Act to some extent limits this right, but there is disagreement about whether it will, in the long run, achieve greater security for children (Rowe, 1975; BASW, 1975). While the sudden separation of foster children and parents is understandably deplored, less obvious is the suffering of the mothers who intended to part with their children only briefly, who may never have been helped to consider the possible long-term future, and who, after many years, cannot bear to relinquish entirely the rights and hoped for rewards of motherhood.

Lambert and Rowe (1973) studied those children who lived in limbo, 'caught in a disabling web of uncertainties and vain hopes'. They were surprised and horrified to find that, in spite of the current emphasis on family care and rehabilitation to their own families, once children under the age of eleven had been in care for six months they had only a one in four chance of returning to their parents. Nearly a quarter of the children studied needed placements in an adoptive or long-term foster home, but there was little chance of this being achieved because of a mixture of the child's characteristics and problems (nearly a half suffered from an illness, mental or physical disability, or had less than average intellectual ability or showed behaviour problems), the supply of substitute parents, the attitudes of social workers and the policies and traditions of agencies. A half of those for whom there was little hope of adequate care were natural children, and it was they who tended to come into care younger, stay longer, and have less contact with their families than their legitimately born contemporaries. Natural children were seldom reunited with their parents, and many of them could have been adopted if their likely future had been recognised and a decision taken earlier. As Parker points out in the preface to this study, although predicting a child's future is difficult, the risks for the child of an endless uncertain wait in care are so great that there is an obligation to make hard decisions in partial ignorance.

Some implications for the counsellor

While it is professionally unacceptable to exert pressure, it is similarly unacceptable to fail to take into account current social conditions and their effects on children's development (Crellin, 1971, p. 112).

The fact that an unmarried mother may distort reality for her own purposes in no way negates the objective existence of that reality; and its impact upon the lives of the girl, and the baby, will be in conformity with the actual facts, not with her fantasies (Young, 1954, p. 175).

Many of the facts about unplanned or unwanted pregnancy, about illegitimacy, about single parenthood and about institutional care, are depressing. They have too often been ignored, not least because of the problems they present for the counsellor (Cheetham, 1976).

Studies of general trends can reveal little or nothing about any single person's future. Many unwanted or natural children, many single-parent families, many people reared in institutions, through a combination of personal qualities, help and luck triumph over all the odds, attain a measure of personal and social competence and a degree of happiness which in no way distinguish them from the rest of the community. There can be no certain predictions about who are the most vulnerable and the most likely to be overwhelmed by a hostile environment.

There are also problems in interpreting the conclusions of research studies. The facts which are amenable to measurement are not necessarily those which reveal an individual's state of mind, contentment or misery. In addition, enthusiasm for demonstrating differences may obscure the evidence. For example, in Crellin's study, while nearly a quarter of natural children were deemed maladjusted, so were 13 per cent of the legitimate. It is also difficult to know how long, with changing social conditions, research conclusions will be valid.

Important though critical scepticism is, it does not justify ignoring the accumulating and largely enduring evidence of the realities of the problems to be faced by most of the people who are the subject of this chapter. Nor does it mean turning a blind eye to the inadequacies of the social services. It is easy for those brought up in the wake of optimistic enthusiasm for the Welfare State to be complacent about its achievements. And complacency may also be defence against the anxiety of acknowledging the full extent of the shortcomings of welfare provisions, particularly when these involve children.

> [Their care] is in any case so emotional a matter, with rivalry between different 'parents' so inevitably present, and the discrepancy often so great between the life of the child in care and what any social worker would wish for his children, that the temptation to avoid looking at the situation as it really is must always be present (Dinnage and Pringle, 1967, p. 31).

People must not be shielded from hard facts. To do so increases the risk of mistakes and deeply regretted decisions. It also weakens the demand for the radical changes in social policy which would protect the most vulnerable members of society.

five

Beliefs, attitudes and facts

The purpose of this chapter is to draw attention to the ways in which beliefs and attitudes may affect the behaviour of those who try to help women who are unhappy about their pregnancies. Just as women's feelings about pregnancy are influenced by their upbringing and education, their experiences of marriage and motherhood, and their perceptions of their roles and their futures, so is counsellors' understanding of women's needs similarly influenced. These emotional subjects become even more complicated to handle when they are linked with beliefs about sexuality and about life and death, the main-springs of our existence. Pregnancy, contraception and abortion, some of the principal themes of this book, arouse our deepest feelings and passionate and confused argument. People who work with pregnant women need, therefore, to be able to distinguish between the help they offer because it fits with their own view of the world, and that which accords more with the objectively determinable facts. And since many of the dilemmas facing women and their counsellors cannot be solved solely by rational argument, this chapter highlights those moral problems with which we must come to terms if we are to be reasonably reconciled to the actions we take.

Sexuality and contraception

It is salutary to recall that the welcoming official attitudes and political enthusiasm for extensions of public provision for family planning in the last few years are the product, not the explanation, of birth control. In this, as in other vital areas of morality, it is the sheep who have led and the shepherds who have followed (Finer Report, 1974, para. 3.15).

The unmarried

Ever since it became possible for men and women to control their fertility by reasonably effective means of contraception there have been debates about the influence this has on the relationships between men and women. Contraception for the unmarried is frequently opposed because of the fear that, freed from the risk of pregnancy, men and women will indulge in illicit sexual relations to an extent which threatens the ordinary conventions of marriage and family life. Since women, rather than men, are seen as the guardians of conventional sexual morality it·is they who, at least publicly, must be constrained from embarking on pre-marital sexual relationships. To this end it is argued that those who offend against the established norms of sexual behaviour may damage themselves psychologically and socially. There is also the fear that promiscuity, often seen as an inevitable consequence of a relaxation of the rules about sexual behaviour, will result in epidemics of sexually transmitted diseases.

On the opposite side, those who wish to promote contraception point out that, whether or not this has been instrumental in encouraging sexual activity outside marriage, it has to be recognised that it is now common for the unmarried to be involved in such relationships either on an experimental or permanent basis. They argue, therefore, that it is only sensible to help people prevent the unhappy consequences of resort to abortion or of giving birth unwillingly to natural children. It is also argued, although perhaps less forcibly, that it is anyway good for the unmarried to have some experience of sexual relationships. This may be seen as the natural culmination of a deep friendship, or as a legitimate physical pleasure, or as an important preliminary to marriage.

Both the proponents and opponents of contraception for the unmarried can draw some support from the known facts. Sexual relationships among the unmarried are now common. These men and women run great risks of pregnancy occurring because they do not use contraception, or because they use it inefficiently (Schofield, 1968 and 1973; Bone, 1973). Abortion is not generally regarded as an acceptable means of disposing with any unwanted pregnancy but as a last resort (Pearson, 1973). The assumption that the unmarried have sexual relationships largely because they are liberated from the fear of unwanted pregnancy therefore seems too simple.

Fears of widespread promiscuity among the young also appear to be much exaggerated. Even those with a very liberated attitude to sex seem to feel strongly that fidelity is essential to a sexual relationship, whether inside or outside marriage. Dating around is acceptable, but sleeping around is not (Schofield, 1968; E. and M. Eppell, 1966; Williams and Hindell, 1972). On the other hand, it is possible that there is a discrepancy between what people say is their ideal and what they actually do (Rains, 1971). It is also possible that there are differences in the attitudes of men (who have been far less studied), and that girls submit more readily to their pressures for casual affairs than they are prepared to admit. It is also true that the incidence of sexually transmitted diseases amongst both men and women has reached alarming proportions.

There seems to be no means of knowing whether sexual relationships among the unmarried contribute to greater happiness than their absence, although common sense tells us that in a society which in many subtle ways extols their pleasures, those not involved may feel in some way deprived. It is also possible that in such a situation people may feel pressured to behave in ways which are not consistent with their religious or ethical beliefs, with all the ensuing conflicts this may mean. It is likely that an individual's conclusions about the implications of the sexual behaviour of the unmarried will be influenced by his or her personal reactions to the strictures and hypocrisy of conventional sexual morality. Envy of the greater spontaneity and frankness that are a part of contemporary life may find expression in condemnation, or in exaggeration of their advantages and disregard of their problems.

Although a general acceptance of the sexual relationships of the unmarried and pragmatic arguments about the prevention of suffering seem to be gaining ground, the related moral problems and the unanswered questions about the implications of such behaviour still exert an influence on contraceptive services and the way these are used, and upon education. The moral beliefs of the members of local and central government plus an awareness of the susceptibilities of their constituents have, until recently, made it difficult for them to support clinics which provide contraceptive advice and facilities for the unmarried. For example, in 1973 in the debates about the provision of free contraception, the then Secretary of State for the Social Services, Sir Keith Joseph, was at pains to point out that he in no way wished these services to represent any threat to family life. The decision a few months later to make contraception available free within the National Health Service 'regardless of marital status and age' certainly did not escape criticism. Some doctors are also unhappy about providing contraception for the unmarried and may feel constrained by legal as well as ethical considerations from treating those under sixteen. Added to this, the doubts of some unmarried people about the legitimacy of their sexual relations may prevent their asking for contraceptive help or using it efficiently (Rains, 1971).

All these fears are compounded by the ignorance about sexuality which is inevitable when the necessary education in human relationships is still largely inadequate. Although it is generally agreed that this education should do much more than impart physiological facts and information about sexual techniques and contraception, there is considerable confusion about its other objectives and the best methods of achieving these. How can young people come to see sexuality in the wider context of human relationships; with what notions of morality for individual responsibility should they be presented? (Ripley, 1969; Schofield, 1973; DHSS, 1974). Although such education probably means a joint enterprise between home, school and leisure centres, spanning several years, little progress has been made with such schemes; not least because of the doubts or embarrassment of the adults who must initiate them.

Married couples

There is today little dispute in Britain about the place of contraception in the sexual relations of married people. Although the provision of contraceptive services has, in the past, been bedevilled by confusions about the ethics of population policies and individuals' right to reproduce, the general acceptance of the significance of sexuality apart from the procreation of children, and of the wish and need for smaller families, has been accompanied by startling changes in attitudes towards contraception, changes which have not yet had time to make their full impact on contraceptive behaviour (Draper, 1972).

At the turn of the century it was widely believed that the practice of contraception would encourage women's infidelity, and by allowing them freedom to regulate their fertility, threaten the very foundations of family life. This fear may still be an obstacle to sterilisation. Less explicitly, freedom from uncontrolled child bearing can be seen as a threat to masculine domination at home and at work. The ability to regulate fertility has certainly been a crucial factor in the movement towards greater equality between men and women.

Only in the last thirty or forty years has the medical profession given its blessing to artificial contraception and political bodies their practical support, not least because, faced with large numbers of abortions, contraception is a much more attractive alternative. Less than twenty years ago a married woman's request for contraception merely because she did not want to have children was frequently not well received. Contraception was intended very largely as a means of spacing children, not as a means of promoting sexual enjoyment, or the freedom to avoid pregnancy altogether (Medawar and Pyke, 1971). A distinction must also be made between the general acceptance of contraception as a normal and desirable part of married life, and active support for services which might achieve this end. There have, until recently, been few efforts to establish those easily accessible clinics or domiciliary services which would make it easier for more women, especially those from the lower social groups, to obtain contraceptive help. There are also deficiencies in the available services (Cartwright, 1970; Bone, 1973). It has not been easy to establish as a priority the necessary finance, premises and facilities, or for contraception to be included in the education of professionals. It is often argued that a couple's sexual relationships are so private and personal that it is their responsibility to ask for contraceptive help and that uninvited professional intervention would be improper or unwelcome. It has also been said that married couples 'find out for themselves' about contraception and that, with the exception of the minority of large families, most seem to control their fertility reasonably efficiently. Taken together these factors account for the fact that a significant number of general practitioners and consultant gynaecologists do not routinely give contraceptive advice (Cartwright and Waite, 1972). However, the incorporation of contraceptive services into the National Health Service may bring significant changes.

The level of service necessary has, therefore, often been defined in terms of the small numbers of men and women knowledgeable and bold enough to ask for help. We know now that these people are in a minority and tend to belong to the higher social groups.

We also know that it is common for married couples to use methods of contraception which are not only inefficient but which also may be a potential source of marital disharmony. And even in small families a child's arrival may be untimely if not actually unwelcome (Cartwright, 1970 and 1976).

Abortion

Some moral questions

Abortion is a far more contentious subject that birth control and likely to remain so. Because it involves the destruction of life it is contrary to many religious and ethical principles. Although abortion has always been widely practised, in spite of stringent civil and religious laws forbidding this, it seems that people have generally been more prepared to condone this illegality, while regretting the obvious dangers of maternal death and ill health, than they are to accept official sanctioning of termination of pregnancy. Arguments about abortion are much fiercer when attempts are being made to legalise it, or in the early stages of a reformed law. In such a situation, attitudes which might best be described as neutral or ambivalent, change quickly to passionate convictions for or against abortion, sometimes because it is feared that official sanctions will encourage behaviour which has previously been only tacitly condoned. Many people in North America and several Western European countries are now caught up in such a debate, and because this involves beliefs about the sanctity of life and the freedom of individuals, facts about the consequences of abortion or unwanted pregnancy do not necessarily change opinions. Nevertheless, profound convictions are no excuse for ignorance. We also need to be clear about our own views of the morality of abortion lest we project our confusions on to those seeking help.

In the arguments about the morality of abortion three main standpoints can be distinguished. The first is that the embryo or foetus is a human person with the same right to life as any child or adult. Such a view prohibits abortion in any circumstances, except possibly to save the life of the mother. It affirms that one person's freedom of the right to abortion is the denial of another person's right to life, and, that any kind of existence is preferable to destruction.

The second view, which is probably the one most prevalent in

Britain, and is characteristic of several Protestant churches, is that the foetus has a moral right to life, but a lesser right than that of an independent person. It may therefore be destroyed to avoid what are considered greater evils than the termination of its life. These views have long been reflected in English abortion law, where termination of pregnancy has commonly been distinguished from other forms of destruction of human life (Hart, 1972).

This approach to abortion usually places the responsibility for decision-making onto medical or socio-medical personnel, who are given some criteria to guide them in their task. For medical as well as ethical reasons the matter is considered too grave to be left to the mother and her partner; experts are required to decide on reasonable exceptions to the general view that life should be preserved. Those who adhere to these principles may also maintain that, since those who cannot assert their own right to life deserve protection, decisions to terminate pregnancy must be taken most cautiously.

The third standpoint maintains that the foetus cannot be regarded as a person at all but only as a part of the mother until it is born, or at least until it has reached the age of viability, which is variously defined as twenty, twenty-four or twenty-eight weeks of gestation. It is therefore maintained that the mother alone should have final responsibility for making a decision about abortion, and that this should be available either on request or on demand. In the first case this means that the woman has to find a doctor who is willing to perform an abortion, although no legal conditions will be attached to such a decision. The second case, that of abortion on demand, is usually interpreted as meaning that, except when there are grave medical contra-indications, a woman has an overriding right to abortion, and that this must therefore be provided by the State.

Those who support abortion on request or demand do so for various reasons. For some the main justification is a conviction that women should have control over their bodies and their own lives and that bearing a child should be their decision and no-one else's. Such a view is often supported by arguments about autonomy and the freedom of individual choice and may draw strength from highlighting the extent to which women's freedom in their sexual and reproductive lives, as well as in their careers, has been limited by the social structure and by male dominance. The right to abortion is therefore an essential component of control over women's fertility, and thus over the pattern of their lives. Others argue that women should bear the responsibility for decisions about abortion, often after full discussion and advice, because any other system is riddled with inconsistency and unfairness. These people point out, rightly, that it is inevitable for there to be considerable differences in the assessments of medical and social conditions and that when individuals exercise their discretion about the interpretation of legal criteria, similar cases are bound to be treated differently. Furthermore, some doctors may be incapable of making assessments which have to take account of social as much as medical considerations. It may also be said that it is wrong to ask doctors to carry responsibility for decisions which may well be as much moral as medical, even though some women may prefer to feel that the weight of the decision has been taken from them.

Underlying these three positions is a debate about the nature of humanity. When does an unborn child achieve the moral and legal status of those who have been delivered from their mothers? This debate, with roots in philosophy, theology, law and medicine, has a long and extremely complex history. It is discussed by many writers including Callahan (1970), Noonan (1970), by the Church Assembly Board (1973) and, more briefly, in volume 1 of the Lane Report. It is only possible here to outline the more important issues.

Those who assert that an embryo or foetus should be treated as a full human being argue that there is no obvious stage in the intra-uterine development when a distinction can be made between a collection of cells, unidentifiable to the naked eye as a baby, and a human infant. They also point out that very early in gestation it is possible to identify human characteristics in a foetus, for instance the heart and other essential organs, and that by ten or twelve weeks the foetus plainly resembles a baby. Furthermore, even before its implantation in the uterus, the fertilised egg contains the full genetic code which will determine its development. From a theological point of view most Catholics and many other Christians maintain that the only logical time to assume that a foetus receives a soul, thus distinguishing it from other living matter, is the time of conception, or possibly of implantation. It is therefore false, it is argued, to make distinctions between potential and actual human life, even when a foetus cannot survive outside its mother's body.

Nevertheless, however illogical it may seem to some people, distinctions are normally made between different stages of gestational development. For example, it is often argued that abortion should not be allowed, or should be much more strictly controlled, when a foetus is viable, that is when it could live, with or without the aid of life-support systems, outside its mother's body. One of the problems of this position, from the point of view of defining legal criteria, is that as medical technology becomes more sophisticated, so the age of viability decreases. And furthermore, what survival rate should justify the reduction of the legal age of viability? For many people there is an obvious difference between a foetus of, say, twelve weeks which, although it may show signs of life after it is delivered, is doomed to die whatever medical care is given, and one of twenty-four weeks which, given this care, has a chance of survival.

There may also be other important considerations. Many women do not *feel* pregnant, even though they may accept this rationally, before they have felt foetal movements. It is common for them to say that, if they are to have an abortion, then this must be before they are aware of a living being inside them. From the point of view of medical staff and the women concerned, the earlier an abortion is performed the simpler it is. The unpleasantness of handling identifiable parts of a foetal body and, even worse, of witnessing the delivery of a complete foetus, is a strong deterrent to abortion. These problems are very largely absent when an abortion is performed early, and particularly in the first few weeks of pregnancy, when it is difficult to identify parts of the foetus or embryo. It can be argued that such attitudes are emotional, and therefore have no place in logical argument. The problem here is that most people's views cannot be divorced from emotion. How we feel inevitably determines how we think, and reprehensible though this may seem, it is usually easier to live with some confusion and ambiguity, than with strict logical consistency.

There are also important debates about the balancing of the rights of individuals and the way such decisions may be made. Some of the most powerful arguments for abortion concern those situations where a mother's life or health is gravely threatened by a pregnancy, where she has become pregnant as a result of rape, or where it is probable that the child will be born grossly handicapped. In these circumstances it has seemed relatively simple, emotionally if not logically, to decide to support the interests of the mother against those of the foetus. Such situations are, however, rare and in those countries where abortion has been legalised, it is common for decisions to be taken in which the health of the mother is assessed in conjunction with her social circumstances, including the health of the other members of her immediate family. If the birth of another child is likely to reduce the quality of life of the family as a whole, is it right that the foetus should be destroyed? And if it seems as if the child's chances of a decent life are small, is it better that it should be aborted?

The answers to such questions will depend partly on how far individuals think it is right to take a pragmatic view, entailing the prevention of suffering wherever possible, and on how far they think that arguments about the quality of life are irrelevant to the principle of the right to life. On the one hand, the ability to control life, primarily by contraception but, if necessary, by abortion, can be seen as an achievement and an essential human responsibility; on the other hand, this may be thought a philosophy of cruelty and despair, possibly discouraging efforts to improve the human lot, since it will prove easier to dispose of those who create problems.

In fact, it cannot be demonstrated that legal abortion leads to a decline in the value of human life, or in efforts to alleviate the hardships of the poor, of the handicapped or of the sick. It is sobering to recall that the worst conditions for mothers and children prevailed when there was no legal abortion, and no means of efficient contraception. However difficult historical comparisons may be, it is generally true to say that at times when abortion has been strictly forbidden, no great attention was paid to the plight of the weaker members of society. Only a hundred years ago it was an accepted fact of life that thousands of children every year would die violent deaths at the hands of their parents, and that thousands more would die or be crippled from malnutrition. For those that survived there was often only a bleak future. Abortion and contraception are only two of the many measures which accompany an increasing awareness of suffering, and determination to relieve it.

Because the moral dilemmas it poses are insoluble it is now common for legal abortion to be supported or condemned more on the basis of its results. The protagonists of both points of view are now engaged in exhaustive and exhausting examinations of the implications of abortion for women and their families, for the medical and nursing professions, and for society (Simms, 1970). What are the comparative risks of morbidity and mortality of abortion and childbirth? Does relatively easy abortion discourage contraceptive practice? Does the need to take part in abortion work affect recruitment to nursing and to gynaecology? Does legal abortion lead to a decline in illegal operations, with all their attendant dangers? Does the availability of abortion lead to a lessening of parental responsibility? It was the task of the Lane Committee to investigate these questions, some of which are easier to answer than others. It is, for example, impossible to establish accurately the extent of illegal abortion. It is also difficult to define and measure parental responsibility. And for how long is it feasible to search for the after-effects of childbirth or abortion?

In its report the Lane Committee tried to indicate those questions which could not be fully answered, either because of their complexity, or because of the present state of our knowledge. However, its general conclusions were that the Abortion Act was working reasonably well, in that it had relieved the suffering of many women and their families. It also concluded that the legalising of abortion had not placed an impossible burden on the health services. The Committee's findings are discussed later in greater detail, and although research has shown some to be beyond dispute, there remain less certain matters. It is, for example, hazardous to relate directly general social benefits or misfortunes to the legalising of abortion. These are more likely to be associated with rising standards of health and welfare, or with general changes in expectations and behaviour. It is also misleading to try and understand the arguments about abortion in isolation. These have to be set in the context of much broader issues, such as the prevailing belief in the right to happiness, or the emancipation of women, or the greater awareness of the fallibility of welfare services. Abortion is likely to remain surrounded by paradoxes, painful to the individual and puzzling for the community.

First opinions are so frequently wrong. The rational man might guess that abortion would be common among poor women with large families; uncommon among those whose religious beliefs teach that it is a serious sin or even murder;

common where it is legal and available in hospitals or clinics and uncommon where it is illegal and punishable by long terms of imprisonment. The rational man might suppose that because abortion involves the destruction of a foetus those who resort to it would be worse parents than those who have term deliveries, and that when abortion is liberally available within a society it might lead to some deterioration in the community sense of social responsibility ... but all these assumptions and many others that a rational man might adopt are profoundly mistaken. In all cases the idea which appears most likely is false and ideas which on a superficial analysis appear to be unattractive are in fact those most likely to benefit the individual and society (Potts, 1973).

Public attitudes

Attempts to assess the attitudes of the public towards abortion and the opinions of women who have been faced with the dilemma of an unwanted pregnancy have been made in two main ways: by public opinion polls and by smaller, more detailed studies which allow the expression of views in greater depth. Both kinds of study are liable to error and to misinterpretation. Questions may be misleadingly phrased to prompt one sort of answer rather than another. When a simple yes/no/don't know answer is required, although the results may be easily quantified, they may give no idea of shades of opinion, which are particularly important in highly emotional or controversial areas. The results of more detailed studies may be difficult to assess in any exact way, and because they may often concern small unrepresentative groups, may anyway be open to question. These studies do, however, illustrate the subtleties of peoples' thinking, their doubts and inconsistencies, and thus provide some indication of how people will actually behave when faced with a complex problem.

Volume 2 of the Lane Committee report summarises the results of most of the large-scale opinion polls on abortion which were carried out between 1962 and 1972. These show that in this decade there was a major shift of opinion in favour of liberalising the abortion laws. In 1971, less than 10 per cent of the population were totally opposed to abortion. Although there are, not surprisingly, differences between social classes, age groups and between men and women, taken as a whole about three-quarters of the population agree that abortion is justified in special circum-stances, and particularly when the mother is, or would become, physically or mentally ill, or when a baby is likely to be deformed. Between 15 and 20 per cent of the population are now said to favour abortion being available 'whenever the mother wants it', and more recent polls show that a majority of electors think that the National Health Service should make special arrangements for abortion and allied services in areas where these are difficult to obtain. However, it is interesting to see that, in spite of these conclusions, the same polls show that a significant number of people, about one-third in some studies and rather more in others, will, if asked, say they think abortion is morally wrong. This response seems to highlight the inconsistencies between moral attitudes and reactions to practical situations.

What do more detailed studies tell us about attitudes towards abortion? Bone (1973) found that in general women considered it an extreme measure, to be used almost exclusively when there were risks to the mother's or child's health, and not for primarily social reasons. Nearly a third said they would not consider having an abortion in any circumstances. However, Bone concluded, from some inconsistencies in the women's replies, that stated intentions about abortion are not necessarily a good indication of future behaviour. It is also interesting to see the extent to which those women who had had an abortion said that their doctors had been responsible for this decision, with many giving the impression that they had had little or no say in the matter. Williams and Hindell (1972) and Cartwright and Lucas (1974), who studied women who had actually had abortions, also found considerable ambivalence about the morality of terminating pregnancies. This was more usually regarded as an unfortunate expediency, although a lesser wrong than bringing up a child in unsatisfactory circumstances, and for single people, in some cases less immoral than constantly being prepared for sexual intercourse by using contraception. Even though almost half of the mothers and fathers studied by Cartwright (1976) thought that abortion should be available on request, the great majority of mothers said they would accept an unwanted pregnancy rather than think of getting an abortion.

Many women said that their opinions about abortion had changed when they found themselves faced with an unwanted pregnancy. Previously they had regarded it as rather shocking and something that 'only happened to other people'. Only a few believed that women should have the right to choose whether or not to have their baby. They were, however, confused about how decisions concerning termination of pregnancy should be made and although clear that 'deserving cases', such as their own, should be sympathetically treated, they frequently did not think abortion should be easily available to certain other groups, for example, the 'promiscuous', or those who could afford to have a child. Abortion was certainly not regarded as a satisfactory form of birth control, even by those who had previously had more than one pregnancy terminated; it was a 'desperate remedy in a desperate situation'.

Perhaps because the moral aspects of abortion seem so important to the women studied, it was common for them to say that any woman considering an abortion should talk it over carefully with an unbiased person. For the great majority, the decision to have their pregnancy terminated had not been easy, and their reflections reveal considerable moral conflict.

> I know it sounds paradoxical but I still have as many moral anxieties about abortion as I ever did which is probably some inborn puritanical thing and I still feel in some way ashamed and that I have got away rather lightly with my own irresponsibility. I would not advocate however that people should be punished for irresponsibility. I am still in a quandary about what to do about telling my parents. . . .
> Also it is a moral decision I had to make with my boyfriend and I didn't feel it was my parents' moral dilemma; it was mine. I would not ever want to have an abortion again – not because of unpleasant experiences but I think abortion does slightly damage one's attitude to the existence of life. I
> know that in order to go through with this abortion I had to shut my mind to things like thinking what the baby would be like (Cartwright and Lucas, 1974, p. 73).

Sadly, little or nothing is known about the attitudes of the sexual partners of the women who have had abortions, partly because it is common to exclude the putative father from any discussion about the pregnancy or the possibility of abortion, and to connive without question if a woman says she wants to conceal the whole affair.

Professional attitudes

The shift in public opinion towards more liberal abortion is also reflected in doctors' attitudes. What is not known is whether this has come about because legalising abortion has made doctors more able to state publicly their private views, or because these have been influenced by a greater awareness of the problems of unwanted pregnancy. Alternatively, are doctors merely finding it impossible to resist their patients' pressures for abortion even though they may be opposed to this? Probably all these factors have been influential.

Doctors' views about termination of pregnancy tend to differ according to their particular fields of practice and their training. Gynaecologists are less likely to feel positively about abortion than general practitioners. For much of their time the former are involved in treatment designed to improve fertility, to lessen the risks of childbirth and to produce healthy infants. Indeed, for many, the obstetrical aspects of their work, the wish to be involved closely in the processes of reproduction and childbirth, provide their greatest rewards. Gynaecologists have always been aware, at some level, of the problems of unwanted pregnancy or of congenitally handicapped children, and many were prepared to perform abortions for health reasons before the Abortion Act. However, because they are not usually involved in the day to day care of women and their families, their problems will have less impact on them than they do on general practitioners or on social workers. Whatever the circumstances of a pregnancy, the safe delivery of a child is usually an occasion for rejoicing, or at least of relief, for the parents and for those who care for them. Faced daily with such emotions gynaecologists inevitably may tend to see only the negative aspects of abortion. And for some, the destruction of life seems the very antithesis of their *raison d'être* and training. Added to this, it is usually gynaecologists who have the responsibility of performing an operation which may be seen either as tedious and technically unchallenging or, especially late in pregnancy, as a thoroughly unpleasant procedure much disliked by supporting staff.

Those gynaecologists who trained some years before the passing of the Abortion Act, when abortion was usually regarded as both criminal and sinful, have had to face radical shifts in attitudes and practice. Few people can react to such profound changes with equanimity, and for many the challenge and heart searching involved are painful. It is therefore hardly surprising that many gynaecologists view abortion work with considerable distaste, seeing it as an operation necessitated largely by human careless-ness, which contravenes ethical principles, endangers relationships with nursing staff and which may adversely affect recruitment to the speciality.

Nevertheless, Waite (1974) found that only 7 per cent of con-sultant gynaecologists had a conscientious objection to abortion and that in certain circumstances, for example when a girl aged less than fourteen became pregnant, or when a pregnant woman contracted rubella, the vast majority said they would terminate a pregnancy. More than half said they would also terminate the pregnancy of a poorly paid working girl or of an unmarried student. A fifth stated they would perform an abortion before the tenth week of gestation for 'whoever requested it'.

Consultants usually take chief responsibility for the assessments of women requesting abortion, sometimes because they believe the legal and ethical implications to be too onerous for junior doctors, sometimes because they fear that these colleagues will be more liberal, and sometimes because they think that their qualified blessing will quell the anxieties other staff have about abortion work. Some consultants are also worried that if they agree readily to perform abortions, this will form the greater part of their referrals, and they will do the work refused by colleagues. The belief lingers on, in spite of the change in the law, that abortion is hardly respectable, and that a reputation in this field will deprive a doctor of more interesting and technically more challenging work. This illustrates the subtle relationship and the complex balance of power between consultants and general practitioners. It is ironic that, in some areas at least, poor com-munication between consultants and general practitioners means that the former are refusing work which general practitioners desperately want done, just because they fear they will be despised for taking it.

These attitudes have a considerable influence on the level of service available to women requesting abortions. This is not solely dependent on the pressure of other gynaecological work or shor-tage of resources. In some areas a high rate of abortion has been combined with an increase in other gynaecological work, very often because abortion patients have been treated early in preg-nancy and therefore the simpler, safer methods could be used (Lane Report, vol. 2, 1974). This early treatment may also depend on doctors' attitudes if lack of sympathy for women with unwanted pregnancies and distaste for abortion can lead to delaying tactics (Cartwright and Lucas, 1974). Doctors less in favour of abortion may also cling longer to the notion that it is always a serious operation demanding long stays in hospital. It may be suggested that although long hospital stays are not strictly necessary from a medical point of view, they can help to bring home to the women the seriousness of abortion. Abortion on a day care basis is sometimes opposed on the grounds that speedy surgical treatment will convey the impression that abortion is a trivial matter, and that unwanted pregnancies can easily be disposed of.

The opinions of general practitioners about abortion have been frequently sought and the results of the various studies are summarised in volume 2 of the Lane Report. Since general practitioners are the doctors most likely to have lengthy contact with their patients and to know their families well their opinions about their medical as well as their social situation are particularly useful. The most recent studies, those by Cartwright and Waite (1972) and the NOP of 1972, found that about 12 per cent of general practitioners had conscientious objections to abortion, and that although roughly a half think the law on abortion should not be changed, between one-fifth and a third favour abortion on request. Between a half and a third wanted more facilities for abortion in their own areas and some of these said they were sometimes deterred from recommending an abortion because of the difficulties of arranging this. General practitioners are more prepared than gynaecologists to recommend termination of pregnancy for primarily social reasons, for example when a poorly paid, unmarried girl becomes pregnant, or for a married woman who already has several children. Although it is not known how many women consult their doctors with anxieties about an unwanted pregnancy, the average number of referrals for a termination of a pregnancy made each year by general practitioners is about seven. Only a very small minority refer more than twelve women a year (Cartwright and Waite, 1972).

Nursing staff are often reluctant to co-operate in abortion work and some have been very vocal in their opposition to the Abortion Act. It is difficult to estimate how widespread this opposition is but the one poll of nursing opinion (Gallup, 1972) found that 3 per cent of nurses refused to be involved in termination of pregnancy. About one half thought that the Act was being interpreted reasonably in their own hospitals, although less than a fifth thought that the interpretation was right in the country as a whole. Between 15 and 37 per cent (the results of the survey are inconsistent), thought that women had a right to have an unwanted pregnancy terminated.

More revealing than these figures are nurses' anxieties about abortion work. Many feel that to be involved in the destruction of life is a negation of their personal and professional principles; and for those who do not have an absolute objection to abortion in any circumstances, there is often little opportunity to discuss with senior colleagues the various reasons for reçommending a termination of pregnancy. It is uncommon for junior nurses to have much experience of nursing in the community and they may therefore be only dimly aware of the many social and emotional pressures on women with unwanted pregnancies. The youthfulness of many nurses can also leave them ill-equipped to cope emotionally with some of the ethical dilemmas outlined earlier. They may therefore feel somewhat exploited, left to care without much support or explanation for women whose needs seem obscure or doubtful. Not infrequently these women may be in a highly emotional state and therefore difficult to nurse. They may also be the source of tension in a ward when some patients, perhaps those being treated for sterility or threatened miscarriage, feel affronted by termination of pregnancy, while abortion patients are, in turn, upset by their rebuffs or moral censure. In these circumstances nurses may co-operate in abortion work reluctantly or resentfully, and only out of loyalty, or obedience, to senior doctors.

Hospitals are hierarchical institutions, much influenced by the attitudes of their consultants. Their smooth running and the care of patients depend to some extent on the willingness of more junior staff to carry out directions promptly and without argument. To the relief, and the irritation, of these staff responsibilities tend to be carefully defined, and nurses are constantly exhorted to respect and trust doctors' judgment, and to co-operate without question in the treatment he has ordered (Menzies, 1960). Thus it is not surprising to find, at least on a superficial level, considerable agreement between doctors and nurses on the ethics and objectives of treatment. It is common for senior doctors to think that they have the willing co-operation of their more junior colleagues whose views about termination of pregnancy are believed to accord with their own. The consequences of such beliefs have been vividly and wittily described by Ingram (1971):

For those in a position of authority [the game of] 'Big White Chief' has been popular and effective. The game is played by a professor or head of department, who imposes on his staff an extreme policy for or against termination. Ostensibly his justification is logical and medical, but covert ethical, religious, and personal motives can often be inferred. The views are enforced in an authoritarian way with all the prestige that the Big White Chief can command, in some cases spreading from patients, staff, and hospital to whole cities and regions. The same view prejudges all individual cases, and decision making is simplified, with a reduction in anxiety. It fosters a complementary game ('Little Indian') among the junior staff of the authority, who say to themselves and to their patients: 'If it wasn't for Big White Chief I could act differently, but. . . .' Big White Chief has far reaching effects. The general practitioner knows his views and will refer or divert patients accordingly; Big White Chief may provoke the provision of advisory services or increase the flow of patients to private services. Within a short time Big White Chief sees only those patients he wants to see and becomes a self-fulfilling prophet (p. 969).

When removed from the constraints of loyalty and obedience it takes little probing of the views of nursing and other staff to find that such a congruence of opinion does not exist. Although they frequently have grave doubts about both liberal and conservative abortion policies, there are few opportunities for sharing these. Junior staff may therefore feel little respected by their senior colleagues, and ultimately less willing to commit themselves fully to their professions and to the 'team approach', the cardinal, if sometimes rather empty, principle of contemporary medical care. Added to this feelings of exploitation, and the strain of work which does not accord with a person's ethical principles, must inevitably affect the quality of care given to patients.

This picture of lack of communication and misunderstanding between doctors and nurses is not universal or static. The education of both is changing to take more account of the social aspects of medicine, and there is a growing awareness of the value of inter-disciplinary discussion. Nevertheless, in some areas tradition and inertia erect formidable barriers to the creation of closer links between different staff within hospitals, and between hospitals and community-based services. Furthermore, the care of women considering an abortion may largely depend on the attitudes of those whose help she is seeking. These attitudes are often not well thought out and can lead to harsh or unfair treatment (chapter 6). What could be done to solve these problems?

The way ahead

The challenge of facts

> Without accurate observations no knowledge is possible, and accurate observation requires emotional freedom to see, even when what is seen contradicts cherished theories (Young, 1954, p. 204).

In emotional situations irrationality may easily prevail; but human beings have the power of reason and can be influenced by facts and by arguments based on these. Many older doctors now say that their understanding of unwanted pregnancy, and their reaction to it, has changed radically as they have learnt more about the facts of sexual relationships, of inadequate contraceptive practice, of legal abortion, of poverty and rising aspirations, and of women's changing roles. This is uncomfortable information because it challenges preconceptions. It may therefore be ignored or held to be irrelevant. Such reactions may partly account for Warren and Carstairs's (1974) finding that, in those hospitals where doctors tended to be unselective in their treatment of requests for abortion, by either agreeing to all or none, there were relatively few requests for reports from social workers. These reports often bring to the doctor's notice information which may not fit well with his decision. While no rational person would agree that it is right for these decisions to be ill-informed, they can be much more difficult when situations are seen in all their complexity.

There is an onus on workers to acquaint themselves with what is known about the general situation of those who seek their help. This knowledge will alert them to the possible vulnerabilities or strengths of individuals, although it cannot be a substitute for exploration of each person's *actual* circumstances. People do not fit neatly into general categories, however useful these may be in providing a broad understanding. We need to know the details of their particular situations, and how they perceive them, because perceptions are themselves facts to be taken into account when assessing needs and offering help. We move therefore from the collection of facts to the study of their relationship to each other, and of the foundation they may provide for explanations about human behaviour.

Theory and hypothesis

There has always been an abundance of theories about human behaviour, many of which are based on moral or theological preconceptions. These may maintain that men and women are motivated basically to do good rather than evil, or that without sanctions men are naturally idle, or that women's sexual and maternal roles render them emotional rather than reasonable beings. It is difficult to test such theories empirically.

Alternatively, theories may attempt to take into account various apparently well-established facts about behaviour. This rational approach probably has more obvious appeal, but it also has many shortcomings. Not enough is known about human behaviour, and about its social and psychological components, to construct a theory which is consistent, and yet flexible enough to account for the infinite variations of individual reactions. We may, however, on the basis of what is known, be able to construct various hypotheses, and these can help to develop and focus our thinking. The risk here is that imaginative ideas can, without difficulty, be accepted as established truths, and that the apparently factual basis of theories is not recognised as inadequate, as merely a disguise for a set of value assumptions. There are no necessary or immutable preconditions of society, of the family or of morality. We must not conclude that what is, must be. Millett's blistering criticism of the consequences of an unquestioned acceptance of certain kinds of social research is a powerful warning.

> Sociology examines the status quo, calls it phenomena, and pretends to take no stance on it, thereby avoiding the necessity to comment on the invidious character of the relationship between the sex groups it studies. Yet by slow degrees of converting statistic to fact, function to prescription, bias to biology (or some other indeterminate) it comes to ratify and rationalise what has been socially enjoined or imposed into what is or ought to be. And through its pose of objectivity, it gains a special efficacy in reinforcing stereotypes (p. 232).

The treatment of unmarried mothers in the last hundred years provides an illuminating example of the dangers of uncritical acceptance of ill-established theories about their behaviour (Cheetham, 1976). A value system which held that extra-marital sexual intercourse was a sin indulged in by weak, wilful or seductive women naturally opted for treatment which would punish, reform or deter. Unmarried mothers were the object of shame and scorn, and were subjected to strict training designed to change immoral 'fallen girls' into chaste and prudent women. The fate of the children of these sinful unions was only rarely considered, and although logically they had to be seen as innocent of their mothers' transgressions, their individual rights and needs were largely ignored. It has to be recognised that such theories prompted both deeply punitive and deeply compassionate reactions.

The movement towards theories which held that the pregnancies of the unmarried were consequences of their psychological and, less frequently, their social problems, spawned various assumptions about the future relationship of the mother and child. For example, by keeping her baby a girl might complete the assertion of her femininity and independence, which, it was held, had led her to become pregnant. Thus the child was seen as having a therapeutic function for the mother, with little recognition of his or her own needs. Alternatively, the problems of unmarried mothers have been seen as so great as to render them unfit to keep their children. While both these assumptions can be true, according to an individual woman's circumstances, they have at times been translated into inflexible theories and become the basis for rigid policies. Noted authorities on maternal health and child care have stated at different times that it is the relatively stable and emotionally healthy mothers who place their babies for adoption or who keep their infants. Workers have been enjoined to design their help accordingly. Not until the researches of Yelloly (1965) and Weir (1970) was it actually known which maternal characteristics were associated with decisions to keep or place a baby for adoption, and their findings on this subject are complex. Furthermore, until about ten years ago little or nothing was known about the outcome for the mother or child of adoption or of remaining together. Ignorance had, however, proved no bar to certain convictions that whatever was being done was right.

The burst of information in the 1960s and 1970s about the

hazards of single parenthood and illegitimacy resulted in less preoccupation with theories about the background to illegitimacy and more concern with the child's future and rights. The needs of children are now being distinguished from those of parents. The next step will be to discover, and then to provide, those conditions of life which would make such distinctions less necessary than they seem today, and to identify, far more accurately than is now possible, those parents and children who will not be able to flourish together.

Experienced workers have seen in their own lifetime radical changes in assumptions about needs and services. It could be argued that a lively awareness that ideologies and theories will change would undermine confidence in their ability to assess a situation and to offer appropriate help. It must be recognised that in our present state of knowledge we are limited to making not infallible, but the best possible, assessments, and to offering the help which seems most likely to fit the needs of each individual, both as he or she defines them, and as they can be determined on other criteria. People need help and decisions have to be made. However, an awareness of the imperfections of our knowledge, the clumsiness of our understanding, and the shortcomings of our services will leave us open to new ideas, prepared for new discoveries, and willing to shape help accordingly. This is the ideal; but it is often more comfortable to remain firmly wedded to unchanging assumptions. How can this complacency be avoided?

Education and training

It is now well accepted, in theory at least, that those concerned with the social, medical or spiritual care of individuals must have an education broad enough to enable them to understand their varied needs, the different influences on human behaviour, and the role of lay and the professional helpers (Todd Report, 1968; Seebohm Report, 1968; Briggs Report, 1972). It is also true that much training is still specialised and narrow in focus, partly because of the short time available to equip people with skills essential to their jobs, partly because the explosion in the behavioural and medical sciences means that there is daily more 'essential' information to be absorbed, and partly because of ambivalent attitudes towards inter-disciplinary co-operation. It is therefore common for nurses and doctors to know little about the day-to-day lives and problems of women with children and to have only a hazy idea of social services. Equally, social workers and lay counsellors may have limited knowledge of difficulties of treating women with unwanted pregnancies and of the medical aspects of abortion.

Experience of work in the community has much to contribute to better understanding of social and emotional problems. This is essential for those who are to be involved on a long-term basis in the care of women with unwanted pregnancies but it cannot be easily provided for everyone. Nor is it always possible to give community-based workers experience of the pressures of hospital work. Workers have therefore to be helped to use their imagination about experiences of which they have no first hand contact. This can be partly achieved by explanation and by lectures which use illustrative case studies, but more helpful are discussion groups and seminars.

Discussion and consultation

An underlying assumption of discussion groups is that the participants learn from each other, and not simply from the nominated teacher or leader. They are therefore encouraged to express their own ideas, to account for these, and to question other peoples' opinions. This method of learning can be helpful when different disciplines, or different grades of staff, feel they are misunderstood or exploited, and have been unable to explain their own attitudes and problems. Inevitably in such groups there will be conflict, and some fear the open expression of disagreement. But conflict which is not properly recognised can be destructive. Hostilities may be expressed indirectly and people may opt out of situations made uncomfortable by underlying tensions. Discussion groups will therefore convey information which might otherwise be inaccessible and prompt understanding of different points of view and alternative priorities. They may also be cathartic. Although perfect consensus and harmony are unlikely to be achieved, greater insight into, and acceptance of, differences can make co-operation easier. The sharing of common problems in discussion groups can also help people identify more clearly the nature of their anxieties and the reasons for inadequate standards of work. Problems clarified are easier to solve (Main, 1971; Millard, 1971).

Group discussion in teaching can also help people to make more objective judgments on the basis of indications or probabilities when facts are not clear. This is particularly important when work is unfamiliar, and when it is influenced by value judgments and emotions. Abercrombie (1960) postulated that judgments might be more valid if there was a greater awareness of the many factors which influence them; in other words, if the process of decision-making were more conscious and accessible. In testing this hypothesis she found that asking medical students to discuss together freely a common task, for example, the diagnoses they would make from X-rays helped them to distinguish between what could be ascertained with available evidence, and what could not, and between real information, that is facts they had obtained directly, and those which they had imagined. The inferences of the students who had joined in group discussions were better supported and more flexible than those of other students. They were also more careful in their use of such concepts as 'normal' or 'average'.

The students were not uncritical of this teaching method. Because it contrasted so greatly with the more formal structure they were used to, it was sometimes accused of being ill-disciplined and time wasting. Ultimately, however, most acknowledged that it helped them to think, speak and listen, and allowed them to share their anxieties about their future roles and responsibilities as doctors. Abercrombie concludes:

> The course demonstrated to the student his own personal
> involvement with his perception of the external world. It
> showed to what an extraordinary extent the information he
> received from any situation depended on his own assumptions
> or preconceptions ... and the authority and the validity of his
> own judgments were questioned ... the aim was to make it
> possible for the student to relinquish the security of thinking in
> well defined given channels and to find a new kind of stability
> based on the recognition and acceptance of ambiguity,
> uncertainty and open choice (p. 141).

Individual consultation, if it involves free-ranging discussion, prompts the clarification of assumptions and is not seen primarily as a forum for giving and receiving advice, is also a valuable means of achieving more thoughtful and objective work. There is now considerable experience, in lay and professional fields, of the help that can be given in this way to people undertaking un-familiar and onerous work (Caplan, 1970).

The elimination of discretion?

Would not the best method of controlling haphazard decisions be to reduce, as far as possible, discretionary powers? Such questions are frequently asked about the process of sentencing, about the administration of social security benefits and about abortion.

The complex arguments about the place of discretionary decisions cannot be examined here. But lest this should be thought a simple matter it should be noted that these raise questions about the balancing of individual and group interests, about the problems of meeting need in unique circumstances, about the criteria for rationing in conditions of scarcity, about public control and individual freedom, and about the weighing of lesser evils. In the context of abortion it is often argued that the destruction of life is so serious a matter that such a decision cannot be left to one individual, and can only be justified if grave suffering will thereby be avoided. Many reformers believe there are advantages in a law which is flexibly enough framed to allow for individual interpre-tation and a changing climate of opinion, but which does not so affront public and professional sensibility that there would be little co-operation with it. By working with such a compromise people are able to contemplate solutions to problems which previously would have scandalised them. When the Abortion Act was passed the medical profession generally welcomed the legal provisions which gave them freedom to exercise their discretion. They resisted then, and have continued to resist, attempts to make them fit their prescription for treatment into largely unworkable categories. Indeed, it was the doctors' feelings that they needed greater freedom to recommend termination of pregnancy than the previous law allowed that led many of them to support the reform of the law relating to abortion (Simms, 1974).

Nevertheless, whilst doctors have the responsibility of recom-mending or refusing abortions it is inevitable that some women, whose circumstances may appear to be similar, will be treated differently. In short, decisions will not be fair in the sense of everyone being treated the same.

If women had the sole responsibility of deciding about abortion there could be no complaints of such unfairness, and some doctors would also be relieved of making decisions which they regard as essentially moral. In spite of many professionals' apparent anxiety to be involved in the moral life of society, there are also Ingram's (1971) 'honest plumbers', who see themselves as essentially technicians, preferring to do what they are told.

Although abortion on request would reduce the problems of decision making, it would not eliminate them. Not all women easily, and independently, make up their own minds what to do about an unwanted pregnancy. Many need to explore its background. Some ask for advice and guidance; not only abortion but adoption and single parenthood may have to be considered. The course of such discussions, and perhaps their outcome, may depend partly on counsellors' perception of needs and the relative advantages and disadvantages of the different ways of helping. Whatever the formal legal situation, they cannot escape the responsibility, and the privilege, of influence.

six

Ways of helping

This chapter examines the help available to women unhappy about their pregnancies. Basic information about the working of the services is included, as well as some indication of their problems and of the difficulties people may have in using them. The intention is to provide counsellors with sufficient knowledge to enable them to discuss the various options available, and to know when to refer people for more specialised help.

Welfare benefits

Many women with an unwanted or unplanned pregnancy face severe, crippling and long-term poverty. This is particularly likely if they are single. Indeed, this prospect, combined with the almost certain difficulties of finding adequate accommodation can turn their unplanned pregnancies into unwanted ones. The welfare benefits available, while providing a bare subsistence income, are usually insufficient to avert this poverty, especially if families are dependent on them for long periods (Hunt *et al.*, 1973; Finer Report, 1974; Young, 1974). But these bleak facts do not excuse counsellors from knowing what benefits there are, and from doing all in their power to ensure that the people seeking their help obtain all their entitlements.

Social security arrangements are extremely complex, and expert advice and assistance may be essential for those unfamiliar with them. This may be obtained from various voluntary organisations, for example, the Child Poverty Action Group, Claimants' Unions, the National Council for One Parent Families, or sometimes from specialist advisors in Social Services Departments. Some addresses are given at the end of this chapter. There are also several useful publications giving details of welfare benefits and how they may be claimed (DHSS Leaflet FBI, 1975; Coote and Gill, 1974; Lynes, 1974; Ashdown-Sharp, 1975; CPAG, 1975). Since these comprehensive guides are cheap and easily accessible only the broad outlines of social security provisions most likely to be relevant to pregnant women are included in this section. Its brevity should in no way be seen as detracting from this subject's importance. Frequently parents' and children's greatest need is for money.

Maternity grants (DHSS Leaflet N1 17A: Claim Form BM4)

This grant of £25 is paid to help with the immediate costs of having a baby. If a baby is stillborn it can also be claimed, provided the pregnancy lasted at least twenty-eight weeks. It is subject to certain national insurance contributions payable by either the woman or her husband. A single woman cannot claim the grant on the insurance of the baby's father. Girls under sixteen are not eligible for maternity grant but they may be able to claim money for a layette and other essential items as a part of supplementary benefits but not until after the birth of the baby. Maternity grant may be paid from fourteen weeks before the baby is due until three months after the birth.

Maternity allowances (DHSS Leaflet N1 17A: Claim Form BM4)

This allowance is available for several weeks before and after a baby is born to women who have been working and paying full national insurance contributions for a certain period (Coote and Gill, 1974; pp. 81-2). The standard rate in 1976 was £8.60 and additional allowance can be claimed by a woman who already has dependent children. The allowance will be reduced if insufficient insurance stamps have been paid, although below a certain number of stamps no allowance is payable. This benefit is not available to women while they are in paid employment. It is normally payable for eleven weeks before a baby is due and for seven weeks after birth. It can be claimed at the beginning of the fourteenth week, and not later than the eleventh week before the expected date of delivery.

Family allowances (DHSS Leaflet FAM 1)

These are cash payments of £1.50 per week for the second and subsequent child in a family. They are paid up to the minimum school-leaving age, or for children in full-time education, up to their nineteenth birthday. There are no contribution conditions for these allowances and they may be claimed by single and married parents. They are treated as part of income for tax purposes and for the assessment of supplementary benefit and family income supplement.

Child interim benefit for one-parent families (DHSS Leaflet CH1B)

This benefit was introduced in April 1976 and will continue until the government introduces the new child benefit scheme. £1.50 per week is payable to the first or only child of a man or woman not living with his or her spouse and not living with anyone else as man and wife. Single parents already receiving certain social security payment, for example widow's pension or widowed mother's allowance, are not entitled to this benefit. The child must either be under sixteen, or under nineteen and still in full-time education. This benefit does not depend on national insurance contributions but is taxable and is taken into account in the assessment of family income supplement or supplementary benefit.

Family income supplement (FIS) (DHSS Leaflet FIS 1)

This is a benefit for people in full-time work (not less than thirty hours a week), who have at least one dependent child, and whose normal gross weekly income is less than the amounts prescribed by Parliament. In 1976, for a family with one child, this amount was £13.50, going up by £3.50 for each dependent child. The amount of the supplement is one half of the difference between the family's normal gross income and the appropriate prescribed amount. The maximum supplement payable in 1976 was £7 per week for families with one child, increasing by 50p for each additional child in the family. FIS is paid for fifty-two weeks, regardless of any change in a family's circumstances. After this period a new claim must be made. FIS can be claimed by single women but not by married women living with their husbands, or by a woman living with a man as his wife. In this case it is up to the husband to claim FIS for the whole family. He will only be entitled to FIS if he is in full-time work. He cannot make a claim on account of his wife's work.

Supplementary benefits (DHSS Leaflet SB1, or Leaflet SL8 and Claim Form B1 for unemployed people)

The purpose of supplementary benefits is to provide income on a non-contributory basis for people who are not in full-time work and whose other income, if any, falls below the level of requirements approved by Parliament. The amount of benefit payable is worked out by taking a person's 'requirements', according to the scale rates, plus an addition for rent, rates and any other additions to which he or she may be entitled, and deducting any other income from the total.

The requirements and income of a married couple in the same household, or of a couple living as man and wife, and those of any dependent children living with them, are counted together. The husband has to claim supplementary benefit for the whole family. Householders, that is people who pay rent for their own homes and buy and cook their own food, are entitled to a higher rate of basic benefit. A young person under sixteen cannot claim supplementary benefit in his or her own right, although a girl may be able to do this for her baby.

In assessing this income the first £4 of any part-time earnings and the first £4 of a wife's earnings will be disregarded. Only £2 of a claimant's part-time earnings can be ignored if he or she is unemployed and required to register for work. Family allowances and income from maintenance payments will not be disregarded.

People over sixteen and fit for work may have to register for work at an Employment Office as a condition of receiving benefit. Mothers with dependent children should not have to do this.

The mother of a natural child may be asked by officials to take out an affiliation order against the father, but they cannot insist that she does this and should not pressurise her. It is not a condition for receiving benefit. The Supplementary Benefits Commission itself can initiate affiliation proceedings, but the woman does not have to reveal the man's identity or whereabouts.

A woman found to be cohabiting with a man as his wife may have her benefit withdrawn as it is assumed that the man should support her and her children, even if they are not his own. There is considerable fear of the 'cohabitation rule', partly because it is difficult to define when a man and woman are actually living together as man and wife. The *Supplementary Benefits Handbook* states:

The existence of a sexual relationship is not in itself decisive and certainly occasional sleeping together does not constitute cohabitation. The fact that a man is contributing to a woman's financial support does not necessarily mean that she is cohabiting with him. On the other hand, if he does not support her financially that is not in itself conclusive evidence against cohabitation (1974, para 18).

An appeal may be made against the withdrawal of allowance on the grounds of cohabitation and while waiting for the appeal to be heard the appellant may apply for payment to be made because she is in 'exceptional need'.

Special weekly additions can be made to supplementary benefit where there are exceptional circumstances, for example when a special diet or extra heating are required. Lump sum payments can also be made for people in exceptional need, for example for someone without essential clothing, furniture or household equipment. Emergency payments may be claimed, for instance, if someone has lost their money or is destitute.

Anyone in receipt of supplementary benefit, or of FIS, is automatically entitled to certain other benefits, for example, school meals, and free milk for expectant mothers and children under school age, and exemption from prescription charges.

The scales for supplementary benefit are fairly complicated and change with rises in the cost of living. For people receiving supplementary benefit for more than two years but not required to register for work, the rates are slightly higher. The most up-to-date information about rates can be found in the DHSS leaflets. The *Supplementary Benefits Handbook* published by HMSO (1974), Lynes's *Guide to Supplementary Benefits* (1974), and the other publications mentioned earlier give details of the special extra allowances to which a claimant may be entitled. These are usually paid at the discretion of officials in the DHSS. Although officials may try to ensure that claimants receive all the extra allowances possible in their circumstances, considerable skill and persistence can be required to discover what is possible, and to pursue a claim. It is here that the assistance of experts can be invaluable, as it may be if a claimant, dissatisfied with a decision on a claim, wishes to go to an independent appeal tribunal. A woman wishing to dispute an allegation of cohabitation may also be well advised to seek this specialist help.

There are numerous complaints about the workings of the supplementary benefits system and although many claimants find they are treated with courtesy and sympathy, this is by no means a universal experience (Streather and Weir, 1974). Some of the difficulties of claimants and of officials have been outlined in chapter 4 and they are discussed at length by Stevenson (1972).

Although claimants may be assessed for supplementary benefits by officials visiting their homes, several visits to offices may be necessary. These can be unnerving experiences for people not used to making claims, and some of those who are also find visits degrading or embarrassing. It can be extremely helpful for such a claimant to be accompanied by a counsellor, or by an expert in the field of social security, if a claim is likely to be complicated. It has been estimated that between a half and nearly three-quarters of unmarried mothers are dependent on supplementary benefits (Hunt *et al.*, 1973). Counsellors who work extensively with these families have therefore a responsibility to understand the details of the system and how it may be used to its fullest extent.

Rent and rate rebates and allowances (DHSS Leaflet FB1)

These may be claimed by people not receiving supplementary benefits who are tenants in either private or local authority accommodation. Rate rebates can also be claimed by owner-occupiers. The amount of the rebate depends on the claimant's gross income (and that of his wife in the case of a married couple), the size of the family and the amount of rent and rates. People with relatively high incomes can get help. For example, in 1976 a couple with three children who paid a rent of £5 a week could earn more than £50 and still qualify for a rent rebate. DHSS Leaflet FB1 provides basic information, but assessing eligibility and amounts of rebate is complicated so the advice of the local council should be sought.

Miscellaneous benefits

Free milk and vitamins are available to:
1. Expectant mothers and all children under school age in families receiving supplementary benefits (DHSS Form A9), FIS, or who are in special need because of low income (DHSS Form W11);

2. An expectant mother who already has two children under school-age, regardless of family income (DHSS Form FW8);
3. All but the first two children under school-age in families with three or more children, regardless of family income (DHSS Form FW9).

Medicines and Appliances prescribed under the NHS can be obtained free of charge by:

1. Children under sixteen;
2. Expectant mothers and those with a child under one year old;
3. People and their dependants receiving supplementary benefits or FIS;
4. People suffering from certain specified medical conditions;
5. Old age and service pensioners.

People not included in these categories but whose income is below a certain level may also be exempt from prescription charges (DHSS Leaflet PC11).

There are similar exemptions for dental treatment and glasses (DHSS Leaflet F11).

Free school meals are available automatically for school-children in families who are receiving supplementary benefits and FIS, and by application to the Education Officer, to children in special need because of their parents' low income.

Educational Maintenance Allowances for children wishing to stay at school after the school-leaving age and assistance with clothing or school uniform may be given to families in need by the local education authority. Social Service Departments are empowered, but not obliged, to give financial and other help to families to prevent children being taken into care (Children and Young Persons Act 1963, Section 1). Departments vary their implementation of this Act and information on local policies should be sought.

Accommodation

Nearly all families with children find it extremely difficult to obtain adequate housing but, because of their social and economic status, for single-parent families the problems are much greater (Finer Report, 1974, vol. 1, part 6). Unmarried mothers are especially vulnerable and about three-quarters live with their parents, often because they have no other option (Hunt *et al.*, 1973).

This section gives only a brief outline of accommodation possibilities. Counsellors who do not have an expert knowledge of the subject are strongly advised to consult the specialist organisations such as Shelter, the National Council for One Parent Families or the Housing Advice Centres which have been established in some towns. This can be particularly important when they are in touch with someone who has difficulties with a landlord, or who fears eviction. Some addresses are given at the end of this chapter. A more comprehensive list can be found in Ashdown-Sharp (1975). The publications already mentioned are also useful, and Shelter publishes a guide to housing rights (Cutter, 1974).

Local authority accommodation

Accommodation rented from a local authority is usually both secure and comparatively inexpensive. However, waiting lists are always long; people with priority claims are likely to have to wait for at least a year before being housed, and waits of five years and more are common. The problems are worst in the big cities, especially London. Authorities vary in their attitudes to single-parent families; some give them priority help and others appear to discriminate against them. A few have special housing schemes for single parents. These vary in quality and there are disadvantages in the segregation of particular groups of people. Nevertheless, anyone needing accommodation is strongly advised to put their name on local authority waiting lists. There is nothing to lose. They also need to be clear about the rules for renewing an application and the implications of moving out of the area covered by the local authority, or into accommodation which will reduce their chances of being housed by a council. Authorities' regulations and policies vary (Ashdown-Sharp, 1975, pp. 207-10).

Local authorities do not have a legal duty to find either permanent or temporary accommodation for homeless families, although they are empowered to do so. They do, however, have a duty to take all possible steps to keep a family together. This may mean offering short-term emergency accommodation in special centres which vary from the reasonable to the dreadful. Alternatively, families may be provided with bed and breakfast in small hotels or boarding houses. There are obvious disadvantages to this type of accommodation, especially for families with children.

Sometimes councils will say that, in spite of the risks and misery of separating parents and children, and the extra expense involved, the only help they can offer is to receive a child into care. While parents can refuse to be separated from their children, they may have no other option and every year thousands of children are received into care because of homelessness. Squatting may be a possible alternative and some councils co-operate with groups of squatters (Ashdown-Sharp, 1975, pp. 229-37).

Private accommodation

Privately rented furnished or unfurnished accommodation is almost impossible for single-parent families to obtain, partly because of the high rents involved and partly because of landlords' discrimination against families with children, especially when there is only one parent (NCUMC, 1973). Private accommodation can also be insecure and checks should be made about conditions attached to a tenancy. A rent book must be obtained from the landlord. If two or three single parents decide they would like to live together, by pooling their resources they may be able to obtain better accommodation than a single family (Ashdown-Sharp, 1975, pp. 210-17).

Housing associations can be the best source of private accommodation, although the waiting lists of many are closed. Like some voluntary organisations they may run special flatlet schemes for single-parent families. These vary in the facilities they offer and in the conditions of residence. Some allow maximum independence in self-contained units, perhaps with a day nursery on the premises. In others there is a measure of supervision and some shared accommodation. A list of housing associations can be obtained from the National Federation of Housing Societies, and of flatlet schemes from the National Council for One Parent Families. It is usually helpful for an application to a housing association or to a flatlet scheme to be supported by a social worker (Ashdown-Sharp, 1975, pp. 218-19).

Some mothers' and children's most urgent need is for short stay accommodation. There is a large number of schemes which include mother and baby homes, flatlets and bed-sitting rooms, with varying rules and objectives. A directory is published by the National Council for One Parent Families. Partly because there is now less social stigma attached to unmarried motherhood, the great majority of single mothers remain in the community or with their parents before and after their confinement. Few wish to go to mother and baby homes, partly because of the restrictions this can involve. Those who do require this accommodation may be the most disturbed and isolated mothers, who need considerable help over and above that of accommodation. This is by no means always forthcoming and the standards of mother and baby homes often leave much to be desired (Nicholson, 1968; Finer Report, 1974).

It used to be common for single mothers to be advised to take residential jobs. This is now generally discouraged by the specialist organisations because of its insecurity and the risks of exploitation and isolation. As a long-term solution to accommodation problems it is usually quite unrealistic. Even when employers are motivated by the greatest goodwill, it is not easy for two families to live together. For residential work to be satisfactory for the mother and her child certain conditions must be met: she must like domestic work to a degree that she can meet her employer's demands, the wages and conditions must be reasonable and she must have privacy and independence.

It should now be clear that single parents' prospects of finding adequate housing are grim. Counsellors must face up to this without becoming totally paralysed by the problems. Finding accommodation needs great persistence and ingenuity. For single parents to embark on this struggle alone can be overwhelming.

Substitute care

Expenditure of time, effort, talent and money on children in need of social care is, above all, an investment in the future. It makes no sense to us, either on humanitarian grounds or in terms of sheer economics, to allow young children to be neglected physically, emotionally or intellectually. By doing so, we not only mortgage the happiness of thousands of children, and the children they in turn will have, but also pile up future problems and expense for society into the bargain (Seebohm Report, 1968, para. 191).

In considering substitute care for their children parents need to know the advantages and disadvantages of all the options before them, and to have some idea of their likely implications for all the family. This is a subject surrounded by myth and prejudices, where firm convictions often prove to be based on shaky evidence.

The effects of substitute care

Substitute care in its various forms has been accused of causing delinquency and other forms of behaviour disturbance and of being an active encouragement of maternal although, interestingly, not paternal neglect. These fears may be the legacy of the dreadful conditions in which children have been cared for outside their homes and which, although now far less common, still persist. They also grow from beliefs that children cannot flourish unless cared for continuously by their mothers. This emphasis on the responsibilities of motherhood may be based on genuine concern for women and children, or it may be 'A new and subtle form of anti-feminism in which men under the guise of exalting the importance of maternity are tying women more tightly to their children than has ever been thought necessary since the invention of bottle feeding and baby carriages' (Mead, 1954b, p. 477). In such a context research findings are frequently ill-digested and misunderstood.

It is Bowlby's pioneering research into the effects of maternal deprivation which is most frequently quoted in criticism of substitute care. Bowlby studied children in institutional care who were separated from their mothers for long periods, and at an early age. Whilst in care many of these children were the responsibility of a changing succession of caretakers, thus making it impossible for them to form relationships of any depth or continuity with an adult. The emotional damage these children suffered led Bowlby to his now famous conclusion that it was essential for mental health that 'the infant and young child should experience a warm intimate and continuous relationship with his mother (or permanent mother substitute) in which both find satisfaction and enjoyment' (1951, p. 11).

Although Bowlby carefully distinguished between partial and total separation, this has not prevented highly general and emotional conclusions about all forms of substitute care being drawn from his work. These conclusions tend to ignore the large amount of later research which has examined, in much greater detail, the whole concept of deprivation, distinguishing between emotional, cultural and physical deprivation, and comparing the differing implications of brief and lengthy separations from parents, of the type of substitute care, and of the age of the child at separation (Rutter, 1972; Bowlby, 1969, 1973).

The most important conclusions of these and other researches into children's development are that they need the attachments which grow from a continuous, loving relationship with an adult, emotional and intellectual stimulation, and good physical care. What might be the ideal or necessary context for such care, or the essential conditions of a 'loving relationship', is far from clear. However, it is now recognised that for social, economic and emotional reasons these cannot be provided by some families, whereas they may be available in well-organised substitute care. Although we can accept as proven the proposition that 'bad' care of children in early life can have 'bad' effects, we need much more careful delineation of what constitutes such deficiencies (Rutter, 1972). We need, therefore, to be discriminating in assessments of the quality of parental, or of substitute, care rather than assume that either is the ideal, or that they cannot satisfactorily be combined.

More relevant to the argument about substitute care, although far less quoted, are the large number of research studies which have examined the implications for children and their families of various kinds of day care (Yudkin and Holme, 1969; Nye and Hoffman, 1963; Wallston, 1973). Taken as a whole these studies are largely inconclusive because of the extreme difficulty of designing research on the care of children with adequate control groups, and with comprehensive follow-up. Children's development and behaviour will be influenced not merely by the fact of their mothers' employment but by features in their home background, by social class, by their parents' personal characteristics, attitudes to work, and the nature of substitute care. Responsible researchers are, therefore, cautious about making generalisations concerning the effects of care outside the home. But it is worth pondering on some of their tentative conclusions.

First, and most importantly, the quality of substitute care is obviously crucial to children's development. They are unlikely to flourish in large groups cared for by a succession of adults as well as they would with constant individual care and stimulus from familiar people. As well as emotional security children need help to develop socially and intellectually. Good quality day care, especially when there is co-operation between parents and staff, has positive advantages for children and their families. That this is generally accepted is evident from the present enthusiasm for pre-school education (Halsey, 1972b; Tizard, 1974).

Second, research shows some relationship between a mother's attitude to work and her children's reaction to substitute care. When work is enjoyed, rather than simply endured, children tend to react more positively. Indirectly this underlines the importance, to her family, of a mother's emotional well-being. It is, therefore, unsurprising to find that the attitude of a woman's husband and close relatives towards her employment may also affect her children's reactions to care outside the home.

Third, there is some suggestion that the regularity of a woman's work may have implications for her children, and that it is preferable for this to be continuous rather than spasmodic. However, an irregular work pattern is often associated with other insecurities within the family, and these, as much as changing forms of care, may influence children's behaviour.

Fourth, some researchers have concluded that the age at which a child begins to be cared for outside the home may be significant, and that greater difficulties arise if this happens before the age of two or three. Numerous government reports have based their recommendations for day care on this assumption (Plowden Report, 1967; Finer Report, 1974). Again, much will depend on the length of separation, the type of substitute care, and on the opportunities for the mother and child to develop a relationship with each other.

Finally, there are claims that children who have experienced various kinds of substitute care in early childhood are more ambitious, more independent and more successful at school than those who never left the care of their parents. Here again other factors in the home may be equally important.

Generalised reactions for or against substitute care are, therefore, highly misleading and potentially damaging:

What is deplorable is that thousands of mothers working outside their homes, who, like many in our survey, are devoted to their children and to their families and have obviously taken great care to see that their children are properly looked after during the time that they themselves are not at home, should be made to feel, as they are now often made to feel, that they are neglectful mothers and perhaps responsible for

untold harm to the future mental health of their children
(Yudkin and Holme, 1969, p. 165).

The possible positive and negative implications of substitute care
for each individual child and family need to be balanced.

Although choice of substitute care may be severely limited by
what is available and its cost parents frequently ask for guidance
in making their decisions. It is helpful to suggest they bear in mind
these questions. What would be the physical surroundings of a
child in a particular form of care? Are there toys and play material
available, and actually used? Is there an outside play area? Are the
children ever taken out for walks? What distances would the child
and parents have to travel? All these questions should be
reasonably easy to answer. It may be more difficult, although
certainly no less important, to find out how long those who care
for the children have been in the job, and whether they intend to
stay. How many children are there? What is their age range, and
are they a constantly changing group? Children form attachments
to each other and it is disturbing to be continuously surrounded by
new faces. It is also helpful for children to have the interest and
stimulus of other age groups.

The most difficult but most crucial questions concern the
'caretakers'' attitudes. Do they expect to form close relationships
with the children in their care? How do they react to parents?
What are their priorities? What kind of regime and discipline do
they prefer? How do the answers to these questions accord with
parents' own ideals?

Information about the different forms of registered and
approved substitute care for children under five can be obtained
from social services departments. A few of these offer parents who
are considering care outside the home a consultative service.

Different forms of care

Care given by relatives

By far the most common form of substitute care is provided by
relatives, usually by fathers. Over 40 per cent of the children of
working mothers are looked after in this way (Hunt, 1968). Advantages of this arrangement are that children remain within
bounds of their own family; it is also usually flexible and either

free or relatively cheap. Disadvantages centre around possible disagreement between parents and relatives about a child's upbringing. These may be especially difficult to handle when a single mother feels a debt of gratitude to her relatives (chapter 4). Ageing relatives may also become less enthusiastic about caring for a toddler than for a baby.

Shared parental care, enabling both parents to have some occupation outside the home, is increasingly being accepted, at least in theory, as both desirable and possible, although the extent of father's actual involvement is unclear (J. and E. Newson, 1965 and 1970; Oakley, 1974b). The necessary flexible patterns of work may well be the privilege of a minority of middle-class couples. Much depends on such practical considerations as a man's terms of employment. How flexible are his hours? Can he work less than full-time? Can the couple, when each works part-time, earn as much as the man on his own? How would such an arrangement affect their promotion? And, while such an arrangement is relatively uncommon, what will the couple feel about the surprise and disapproval they may encounter? Have they been able to work out their priorities about work and the care of children so as to avoid later resentment and misunderstanding because shared care will have profoundly important implications for their perception of themselves as workers, as wage earners and as parents. If shared parental care was to be seriously accepted as a worthwhile pattern of life it would involve profound changes in assumptions about male and female roles.

Nannies and mothers' helps

Very few families can afford, or have sufficient accommodation for, living-in help, but when this is a practical possibility it can have several advantages. Children remain in familiar surroundings with people whom they get to know well, and who may become accepted as part of the family. The main problems of such arrangements concern misunderstandings of the respective roles of parents and 'helps', and the tensions that can arise when people live in a family without belonging to it. Those contemplating this form of complementary care need to ask themselves what they expect from living-in help, what rewards there will be for such a person and how they will react to someone else living in their house. If they are employing a foreign girl as an *au pair* will the work they want her to do allow her sufficient free time for her own pursuits, because it will be on this understanding that she takes the job? Are they prepared for the possible homesickness of such a girl? In short, are they willing to take some responsibility for someone, possibly foreign, and perhaps in her first job, who may not be fully mature and who needs the support of family life?

Because there tends to be a high turnover among living-in help parents also need to consider carefully the responsibilities they expect such people to have for their children. If their role is essentially a complementary one then children may not be too disturbed by fairly frequent arrivals and departures. But these changeovers can be confusing and upsetting for children cared for almost entirely by a mother's help, especially if her English is poor.

Day nurseries

Day nurseries usually accept a child a few weeks after birth and, if they are run by a local authority, charges are related to parents' income. Private nurseries run in conjunction with industrial firms or service organisations, such as hospitals, are usually subsidised. If they are not, the fees are usually well beyond the means of most working women. Although day nurseries are open for relatively long hours it is unusual for them to cater for early or late shift work.

There is a high demand for day nursery places and considerable variation in their provision. Although on average there are about five and a half places for every thousand children under five, about fifty local authorities have no places, whereas a few have considerably more than the average. Places tend to be reserved for families with special need, or for the children of parents with 'essential' occupations. All day nurseries have long waiting lists and it is estimated that by 1983 they will still only be able to cater for about 7 per cent of the under fives in single-parent families (Finer Report, 1974).

Day nursery regimes vary. While all provide good physical care, the environment of some may not be particularly stimulating. The total number of staff and children may also be large, although they are usually divided, for at least part of the day, into smaller groups. Staff turnover can be high, and depending on their background and training, some find it hard to make easy relationships with parents, who may in turn feel inhibited by a nursery's atmosphere of expertise and efficiency. However, these experiences are not universal. There are, for example, some nurseries run in conjunction with nursery schools where there is a greater willingness to involve parents, many of whom are greatly helped by the staff.

Nursery schools

Nursery schools cater for children aged between three and five, and are now generally accepted as a valuable, and for some children, an essential prelude to primary education. Their standards are usually high and by long tradition their work is based on an appreciation of the child's social, emotional and intellectual needs. Since the majority of nursery school places are part-time and the school year and school day do not coincide with adults' normal working hours they cannot usually be of much assistance to parents who are working. Nevertheless, demand for places is high and mothers are not criticised for sending their children to nursery school, as they tend to be when they use other kinds of substitute care.

Only about 6 per cent of children receive State nursery education; about twice this number are catered for in private establishments. Places in local authority schools tend to be reserved for the most desperately needy children and in many areas it is quite impossible for children from two parent families, with no acute problems, to receive nursery education unless their parents can pay for this. In 1972 the government said it intended to increase very substantially the number of nursery school places during a ten-year period, making nursery education available to nearly all four-year-olds and half the three-year-olds. It is highly unlikely these targets will be achieved at a time of economic stringency.

Playgroups

The playgroup movement has gathered remarkable momentum in the last decade and now caters for about a quarter of a million children aged between two-and-a-half and five years. The movement had its origins in middle-class parents' growing awareness of their children's needs for social contacts and stimulating play, outside their homes. The dire shortage of nursery education prompted these self-help groups. They have now come to be accepted as a valuable means of helping deprived children and are thus supported by statutory and voluntary welfare organisations. Since playgroups either depend on, or encourage, the participation of mothers there may also be a means whereby mothers can make contacts outside the home and become more aware of their children's potential and how their needs can be met. In short, playgroups can help parents enjoy their children more.

Since playgroups usually run for a few sessions a week only rarely can they provide substitute care for a child whose mother works. Their hours, and in some cases their ideology, are not geared to this. They are, however, sometimes used as an adjunct to child-minding services, thus enriching the play of children cared for in these circumstances.

Child minders

By law anyone, other than a close relative, who cares for a child outside his or her own home for reward, for more than two hours a week, must be registered with the local authority. Registration depends on an assessment of suitability to care for children and on the facilities available in that person's home. There are regulations about fire safety, the ratio of space to the number of children who can be minded. After initial registration child minders should be visited by local authority representatives to ensure that the care being given meets minimum standards.

In 1973 about 57,000 children were cared for by registered child minders in circumstances ranging from excellent to barely adequate, depending upon the standards of the local authority, the local pressure for substitute care and parents' income. At one extreme children may go to a minder whom they know well for a few hours a day. Parents and minders may both be fully involved in their care and regard this as a joint enterprise. The care provided may consist of far more than the somewhat mechanical and routine aspects suggested by the term 'child minding', and be fully geared to children's developmental, social and emotional needs. There will be all the advantages of being cared for as one of a small group of children, in a homely atmosphere. By contrast there are unfortunate parents whose hours of work are so long and irregular that their children spend the major part of their life with minders who, working extremely long hours for small financial reward, may lack the energy and impetus to provide more than the minimal care which should be ensured by registration. As one of the consequences of their parents' search for any, or for improved, accommodation and employment these children may also experience frequent changes of child minders. But probably the most vulnerable children are those placed with unregistered child minders, and for every registered minder there may be ten who are not registered (Jackson, 1976).

Child minders may fail to register for many reasons. Some may be ignorant of the law. Some may resent the intervention of officials. Probably most do not register because of fear they would not be acceptable to the local authority, either at all, or for as many children as they would like to take.

It would be wrong to think of these women as viciously exploiting parents' needs for substitute care, while deliberately neglecting the children in their charge. Although some children are cared for in dreadful circumstances it is more common to find women aware of parents' urgent need for care and willing to help them out, often for very low charges. Sometimes unwittingly, sometimes because there seems to be no feasible alternative, these women may neglect their charges' physical and emotional needs. In their desperation parents may be tempted to turn a blind eye to these shortcomings, and even when they are aware of them there is often no possible alternative (Community Relations Commission, 1975).

These unregistered child-minding services are bound to flourish while there is a desperate shortage of nurseries and nursery schools. Some local authorities are now abandoning punitive policies of detection and prosecution for a programme of advice, practical assistance and training. Many registered child minders would also profit from this help and it is urgently needed if the quality of the only major system of substitute care for working-class children is to improve. It is also suggested that the state should pay suitable child minders a minimum salary as a contribution towards the improvement of services, and in recognition of the extreme importance of providing high-quality care in the pre-school years.

Foster care

The most drastic, and for the majority of parents probably the most unpopular form of care, is fostering, either privately or through the local authority. Children may be placed with foster parents on a weekly basis, but more commonly continuously, until their own parents are in a position to provide care themselves. This may take weeks or years, and the longer the period the more likely it is that foster parents come to be seen as the most important people in a child's life. Indeed, a child placed very young with foster parents may find it impossible to form a real relationship with his natural parents.

For most young children foster care has long been accepted as preferable to institutional care. Its obvious advantages are that it provides the opportunity of close and continuous attachment to parental figures and life in an 'ordinary family'. It also has many inherent problems, not always obvious to those who believe that children will flourish anywhere given reasonable physical care and the kind hearts and good intentions of those responsible for them (Trasler, 1960; Parker, 1966; George, 1970). The relationship between natural and foster parents is inevitably a delicate one and can bring many difficulties. How do foster parents keep alive a child's attachment to adults he rarely sees, especially if they are regarded as inadequate parents? How do natural parents react to their child's growing relationship with his foster parents and their apparent exclusion from his world? Moreover, it cannot be assumed that foster children automatically find a place in their new homes. Their previous experiences may have left them emotionally deprived or difficult to handle, and the easiest child may prove an unacceptable rival for foster parents' own children. In addition many foster parents have to live with the fear that the children, in whom they have invested so much, may be taken from them.

Social service departments select foster parents with considerable care and provide supervision and supportive services. However, these safeguards apply very largely to children in their official care, children are usually only received into care if their families are quite unable to provide for them. It would be most unusual for a local authority to take into care the child of a single woman whose chief reason for requesting this was her wish or need to work or study. Similarly, a child whose parents are living together, and on good terms, will rarely be received into public care, except as a very temporary measure, or because of homelessness, whatever the reason for requesting foster care.

These policies are based on the belief that the long term interests of both children and parents are better served if they remain together. It is also thought wrong for public bodies to appear to undermine parents' responsibilities for their children. Local authority residential child-care services are intended for crises, to be used as the last resort.

These policies do not deter desperate parents, and when day care services are not available, the only alternative is private foster care. Paradoxically, policies intended to protect children in fact frequently result in their receiving care of a most dubious quality, with minimal supervision being exercised by the local authority. Although the majority of private foster parents are well-intentioned kindly people, with some awareness of the special needs of foster children, many are nevertheless at serious risk of emotional and educational deprivation, partly because of experiences prior to fostering, and partly because of serious shortcomings in the care provided. Private foster children are also vulnerable because they tend to be very young when separated from their parents and to experience short stays in a variety of foster homes. Many have little contact with their natural parents (Holman, 1973).

The selection of private foster parents, and their agreement to take a child, are very largely private arrangements between the people concerned. While this has obvious attractions for both parties there are also many risks. Choosing someone to care for children, especially when parents are under stress, is a complex task, and the choices may anyway be extremely limited. Although social service departments have a duty to supervise private foster homes their powers are limited and they are little involved in decisions about placements or selection. Uncertainties about their role and pressure of work may also mean that their supervision is minimal. This may alter with the Children Act 1975. Social workers are disturbed by these shortcomings and the fact that shortages of alternative sources of substitute care can lead them to conclude with unsatisfactory private foster placements.

While it is unlikely that counsellors will meet many parents for whom foster care is their preferred form of substitute care, there are some for whom this may become inevitable, and a few whose cultural traditions may mean that they tend to stress the educational and social advantages of fostering, and to be less aware of its potential hazards. Counsellors have therefore a difficult and painful task. Although parents may be in great distress, and their options few, they need to consider the hazards of fostering. They may be well advised to seek expert social work help. If so, they need some understanding of the working assumptions of social service departments and to be prepared for rebuffs if requests are made which are thought irresponsible or inappropriate. The plain fact is that if a local authority refuses to receive a child into care, and the natural parents resort to private arrangements, no one may receive much help from social service departments. These departments do not wish to be unhelpful. Like their clients, they are victims of gross inadequacies in resources. These are, in part, the result of inconsistent attitudes in society, which while they demand that children should be adequately cared for, do not approve the means to make this possible.

Sadly, it is unlikely that there will be radical changes in the policies affecting substitute and complementary care while this is seen largely as a response to social problems. Significant improvements could only be achieved if it were widely accepted that such care has a positive contribution to make in meeting the needs of children, both directly as a worth-while educational experience, and indirectly by lightening the burden on families, and particularly on mothers. There is at present a basic incompatibility between successive governments' apparent commitment to continued female emancipation, their policies for nursery education and their collusive toleration of low-standard child-care services. There is still a long way to travel from the gloomy resignation echoed by the Plowden Committee less than ten years ago. 'Much as we deplore the increasing tendency of mothers of young children to work, it would be unrealistic not to count its economic yields.' Working mothers need to be seen as more than a buttress to the nation's economy. If women are forced to make absolute choices between motherhood, further education or employment, increasingly unplanned pregnancies will be unwanted, and mothers will doubt their capacity to care adequately for their children without regrets, or resentment, or an undermining sense of failure.

Adoption

Adoption is a subject on which many people feel deeply and are apt to hold somewhat biased views. It touches many sensitive areas of life and often an individual social worker's experiences has been limited to one aspect of an adoption service. This might be the anguish of unmarried mothers in the maternity ward, the happiness of adoptive parents receiving a longed for baby, the problems caused by adoptive breakdowns in adolescence, or the satisfactory adoption experience of a relative or friend (Association of British Adoption Agencies).

Parents who are clear that they wish seriously to consider placing a child for adoption should, as soon as possible, seek the help of an agency which offers a comprehensive service to parents and children, including adoption facilities. Such an organisation could be a social service department, although not all at present act as adoption agencies, or it might be a voluntary society. The Children Act 1975 requires all local authorities to provide a comprehensive adoption service but this part of the Act has not yet been implemented. Information about these agencies can be obtained from the Association of British Adoption and Fostering Agencies.

Far more common are parents who either know little about adoption, or think it immoral (chapter 4), or who, fearing the intervention of officialdom and of losing control over their own lives, dismiss this option without serious thought. It can, therefore, be helpful for there to be some preliminary and informal discussion about adoption, together with the other alternatives that need to be discussed when pregnancy is unwelcome. Apart from basic information parents may need to reflect on their reasons for feeling so antagonistic to adoption. Greater clarity about this can help their other decisions.

Some counsellors are unwilling to broach the subject of adoption, possibly because of their own strong feelings about this, or because they prefer to accept unquestioningly a girl's statement that 'she could never give her baby away'. Understandably they may be deterred by the complexities of adoption. Although they cannot give expert help, if parents are unwilling to approach specialist agencies, as they usually are, there may be no other opportunity even to consider adoption. Natural fears of appearing to be pressurising someone to part with a child can also inhibit discussions, although the presentation of different possibilities need not, if done sensitively, be seen as persuasion that any particular one is the ideal.

Adoption and the law

The Children Act 1975 has substantially changed the law relating to adoption. Not all the Act's provisions are yet in operation and although the following sections outline the existing as well as the new law, the complexities of this mixture of procedures means that counsellors, and those seeking their help, should obtain expert advice on legal matters.

By legally adopting a child the adoptive parents assume all the rights, duties and obligations of his natural parents or guardians. They become as responsible for the child's maintenance and education as if he had been born to them as a married couple. It follows, therefore, that on the making of an adoption order, the child's natural parents lose these same rights and responsibilities. Under the Children Act 1975 adopted children over the age of eighteen may obtain a copy of their original birth certificate.

There are about 20,000 adoption orders made every year. Only about half of adopted children are adopted by people unrelated to them. The rest are adopted by natural parents, most usually after their marriage to each other, or to someone else, or following divorce and remarriage. With the implementation of the Children Act 1975 this situation will probably change because it will become more difficult for parents and step-parents to adopt if the natural parent has been divorced and remarried. Courts will, as an alternative, have the power to make a custodianship order in some cases of proposed adoption by a relative.

Under the Children Act 1975 adoptions can only be arranged by registered adoption agencies (including social service departments), except when the proposed adopter is a relative of the child. Arrangements can then be made independently. However, this part of the Act is not yet operative and until it is children may still be placed for adoption by private individuals. It is generally agreed that there can be grave risks attached to such procedures (Houghton Report, 1972).

Consent to adoption

Although a mother may have decided during her pregnancy, or shortly after she has given birth, that she would like her infant to be adopted, she cannot formally give her consent to adoption until the baby is six weeks old. Consent may be given in respect of a particular adoption or, under the Children Act 1975, the parent can agree to 'free a child for adoption', in which case the adoption agency assumes parental rights and duties on the understanding that an adoptive home will be found. Under this procedure, which, at the time of writing, is not operative, parents can choose whether or not they wish to be informed by the agency about the progress of the child's adoption. If no adoption order has been made after a year, and the child has not been placed with prospective adopters, parents may apply to the court for the original order to be revoked. Under the new procedure a parent who is agreeing to an order freeing a child for adoption may withdraw the child any time before the hearing, although this may not be done after an application for an adoption hearing has been made and when the court is being asked to dispense with parental agreement. Under existing procedure a parent may not remove a child from the prospective adopters without leave of the court once an application for adoption has been lodged.

In decisions about adoption a court must give first consideration to the need to safeguard and promote the welfare of the child. Before an adoption order is made it also has to be satisfied that every person whose consent is necessary has consented to, and understands, the nature and implications of an adoption order. This order cannot be made until the child is at least nineteen weeks old and has been continuously in the care of the prospective adopter for at least thirteen weeks. However, with the new procedure a mother may, if she wishes, finalise her part in the adoption process any time after the child is six weeks old. With the adoption of a child of a married woman, when the woman's husband is not the father of the child, courts vary in their attitudes towards obtaining his consent. Some courts insist he must be contacted while others do not. Local adoption agencies usually know the practice of their courts.

If a mother is unmarried, only her consent to adoption is necessary. The consent of the natural father is not required, even if he has maintained the child, although in this case he has the right to be informed of the adoption. He also has a right to apply for custody of his child. This application might delay the adoption process, and prevent it if he were successful and refused to consent to the adoption. Such applications are rare. However, if a father has custody of his natural child by an order made under the Guardianship of Minors Act 1971 his agreement to the adoption will be required. Despite natural fathers' limited legal rights, it is increasingly the policy of adoption agencies to involve them in decisions about their children.

Parents' consent can only be dispensed with if they have abandoned, neglected, persistently or seriously ill-treated the child, or have failed, without reasonable cause, to discharge parental duties, or cannot be found, or are incapable of giving consent, or are withholding consent unreasonably (Children Act 1975). Courts have varied in the stringency with which they have interpreted this power to dispense with parents' consent but there is some evidence that they are now doing so more freely.

Adoption procedures

While an adoption agency may try to find an adoptive family with the characteristics favoured by the child's natural mother, the mother will not usually meet the prospective adopters or know who they are. They are likely, however, to be told something about each other's backgrounds.

It used to be thought that only children from a European background, whose parents had no inheritable mental or physical handicap, would be acceptable for adoption. This is not the case today and the general shortage of babies for adoption, plus greater skill in arranging this, mean that most children, including the handicapped, should be able to find an adoptive home, particularly if this is sought in early infancy.

Probably the factor most likely to impede arrangements is the natural mother's uncertainty about the adoption. In the interests of both the child and the prospective adopters agencies are reluctant to arrange adoptions if they think the mother will change her mind before the final order is made. However, it is well recognised that some will need a few weeks after birth before they can make a final decision about their infant's future. For this reason short-term fostering is often arranged although this should not be seen by the mother as a way of avoiding, over a long period, reaching a final decision (chapter 4, pp. 82-4).

Some women say that once they have seen or nursed their babies they know that, whatever their original intentions, they will be unable to give them up. These feelings must be respected and a mother should never be forced, against her will, to nurse her infant. To make a woman do this may be severely limiting her freedom of choice about adoption, becuase the prospect of parting becomes too painful (Raynor, 1971). Other women may be reassured by this brief opportunity to care for their infants (Bernstein, 1966).

The results of adoption

The problems of follow-up and of obtaining adequate control groups make it difficult to study the outcome of adoption. For example, if in adulthood people who have been adopted are found to have considerable problems of relationship and identity, what conclusions should be drawn? It would be mistaken to take this unhappiness as evidence that adoption was wrong for them without knowing whether the alternatives would have been better. It is also possible that these adults' problems could have been more skilfully managed (McWhinnie, 1967). Nevertheless, the most comprehensive study of children brought up by adoptive and natural parents showed that, on the aspects of attainment measured adopted children, at seven-years-old, did better than their peers (Crellin, 1971: chapter 4, pp. 74-8). It is not yet known whether these achievements are maintained in adolescence. The adoption of older children also seems to be reasonably successful, especially when compared to long-term foster care (Jaffee and Fanshel, 1970; Kadushin, 1970). Less conclusive are the numerous studies of the implications of adopted children and parents' background, and of various aspects of adoption practice (Kellmer-Pringle, 1966).

Studies of the factors which predispose a mother to offer her baby for adoption suggest that girls from disturbed or poor social backgrounds are more likely to keep the infants. This may, in part, be a consequence of inadequate social work help (Vincent, 1961; Yelloly, 1965; Weir, 1970).

Practically nothing is known about the reactions of mothers whose children have been adopted, but existing evidence is somewhat sobering. Although women considering adoption receive considerable help during their pregnancy and before they have parted from their baby, after separation, inevitably a time of grief and mourning, there tends to be little contact with social workers (Weir, 1970; Triseliotis and Hall, 1971; Raynor, 1971). These mothers need to be helped to see adoption as giving to their children the best possible home and future, not as giving them away. Allowing a child to go to an adoptive home can thus be perceived as an expression of good parenting. Many women lack this support at the time they most need it.

Both the facts and uncertainties of adoption highlight the heavy responsibilities of balancing the happiness and interests of one person against another. While there is some comfort in Rowe's (1966, p. 49) assurance that a wrong decision for the baby cannot be a good one for the mother, a good decision for the child can be painful and damaging to natural parents (Cheetham, 1976).

Abortion

Abortion has always been regarded as a solution to unwanted pregnancy, although only in about the last fifty years have changes in law and medical practice begun to remove it from the shadow of secrecy and criminality. In Britain induced abortion as a legal form of medical treatment, given certain conditions, has been available for less than ten years. It is therefore not surprising that, while everyone knows something about abortion, it may still be a taboo subject, arousing fears of unsavory practices and of pain and risk to women. By contrast, partly as a reaction to such views and strenuous efforts to educate professionals and the general public, it is not uncommon for therapeutic abortion to be represented as a trivial and completely safe procedure.

The Abortion Act 1967

The Act is permissive in that it states that a person will not be guilty of an offence when a pregnancy is terminated by a doctor when two medical practitioners are of the opinion, formed in good faith, that:

(a) The continuance of the pregnancy would involve risk to the life of the pregnant woman, or of injury to the physical or mental health of the pregnant woman or any existing children of her family, greater than if the pregnancy were terminated

or

(b) There is a substantial risk that if the child were born it would suffer from such physical or mental abnormalities as to be seriously handicapped.

In determining risks to the pregnant woman's health account may be taken of her 'actual or reasonably foreseeable environment'. This is sometimes described as 'the social clause' of the Act, but the law only allows a woman's social circumstances to be taken into account in so far as they affect her health. They cannot, on their own, be considered as grounds for an abortion. An abortion must be carried out in a National Health Service hospital or licensed premises. The Act also states that no one with a conscientious objection to treatment authorised by the Act should be required to take part in it.

These criteria for termination of pregnancy can be interpreted in very different ways depending on a doctor's definition of health and risk. There are a few doctors who will abort any woman before the twelfth week of pregnancy, if she requests this, because statistically the risks of mortality associated with childbirth are greater than those associated with first trimester abortion, the risks being slight in each case. Most doctors interpret the Act less liberally, and a few will only abort a woman when they believe her health will suffer very seriously if the pregnancy continues, or when they are sure that the child will be severely handicapped. This difference of interpretation of the Act is one factor affecting the availability of abortion in National Health Service hospitals and the development of private services. These now cater for nearly half the women resident in the UK, either because they prefer the extra privacy and comfort this may mean or, much more commonly, because they find that only by paying will they be able to obtain an abortion.

Ways of obtaining an abortion

Counsellors should try to ensure that the treatment women receive will be sufficiently comprehensive to meet not only their medical needs but to take account of any social and emotional problems they may have.

General practitioners are well placed to provide such a service, especially if they already have some knowledge of a woman and her family. They can arrange for her to have a reliable and free pregnancy test, an essential first step in diagnosis. They may also be able to provide counselling, or if they feel unequal to this, or a woman appears to have special needs, refer her to a health visitor, social worker or psychiatrist. It is rare for a woman to obtain an abortion in a National Health Service hospital without being referred by a general practitioner. Most general practitioners also know where women can receive good private treatment should this seem the most appropriate, or the only way of obtaining an abortion. Finally, they can provide or arrange any short- or long-term after-care a woman may need. Cartwright and Lucas (1974) found that general practitioners were the first professional people consulted by the great majority of women who had had an abortion. They were then usually referred to gynaecologists in hospital or clinics. Only a small minority saw a psychiatrist.

Those women who are not registered with a general practitioner, or who are unwilling to consult one, or who are dissatisfied with the treatment they have received, most commonly turn to the private sector. Women may also decide to seek private care if they encounter long delays in obtaining hospital treatment. Although it is possible to transfer to another general practitioner, many women are unwilling to pursue this alternative, partly because the procedure can take some time, and anyway requires the consent of the first general practitioner, and partly because they may not know where they will receive more sympathetic treatment.

Most private treatment for British women is provided by non-profit-making organisations such as the British Pregnancy Advisory Service; they now arrange the abortions of about two-thirds of these private patients (Lafitte, 1975). Voluntary services usually provide free pregnancy tests, an initial consultation, which includes a medical examination and counselling, and they can arrange for abortions to be performed in their own clinics. They also offer help with contraception, including sterilisation. At the time of writing the charge for a consultation was about £10, and an abortion for a woman less than thirteen weeks pregnant costs between £50 and £60. The charges are higher for a pregnancy of longer duration. Loans and some free abortions are given to women who cannot afford these charges.

The great majority of women consulting these non-profit-making organisations have abortions. This is a reflection partly of their staff's liberal interpretation of the Act and partly, no doubt, of the fact that many of the women approaching such organisations have definitely decided they want an abortion, and therefore go where they think this is most likely to be obtainable. The counsellors employed by these organisations try to make sure a woman really wants an abortion, and they certainly should not put any pressure on the person who is undecided. They may not, however, discuss in detail all the alternatives available unless specifically asked about these. When an abortion has been arranged a woman's general practitioner is usually informed, but this will not be done if a woman does not agree.

Women can refer themselves to these organisations. Referrals are also made by doctors, social workers, some family planning clinics and agencies such as the Brook Advisory Centres, and Release, which will also help a woman obtain an abortion in National Health Service hospitals where this seems feasible. Since there are some variations in the services offered by non-profit-making organisations the counsellor should find out what these are before making a referral. Lafitte (1972, p. 9) fairly describes the limitations of voluntary organisation;

> Even the finest conceivable voluntary abortion service can have only a brief contact with its patients; it can give them only a small number of specific services when they may need many; and it is usually unable to follow them up. But a decisive shift of private abortion work into the private sector requires large changes, particularly in attitudes in the NHS and particularly in its hospitals.

Abortions can also be obtained in clinics run as profit-making concerns whose fees are higher, and frequently much higher, than those of a charitable agency. A woman less than thirteen weeks pregnant may be charged between £80 and £200; after this period she may have to pay up to £500. Referrals, either directly to the clinics or to the doctors who will perform the abortions, are made by the general practitioners but more usually by the commercial pregnancy advisory services, whose titles, for example, Pregnancy Advisory Bureau or Pregnancy Information Centre, are often similar to those of the non-profit-making organisations. These agencies vary in the services they offer. They may provide consultation with doctors willing to perform abortions, or merely information about which doctor or clinic to approach. Some organisations also include pregnancy testing and help with contraception. Some highly disreputable pregnancy advisory services have been responsible for much of the exploitation of women seeking private treatment. The Department of Health and Social Security now publishes a list of approved fee charging referral agencies which offer a reasonable standard of service. They will, however, remain more expensive than the non-profit-making organisations and should be avoided whenever possible. If there is no alternative but to refer a woman to a commerical agency, and this frequently happens when foreign women are seeking an abortion, stringent enquiries should be made about the exact nature of the services provided and the fee.

In helping a woman decide where it would be most appropriate for her to try and obtain an abortion the counsellor has to balance her own needs with what is known of the resources within her reach. Both public and private services have been justly criticised and praised, according to the needs of the women seeking their help and the variations in their facilities. Crucial factors to bear in mind are the duration of the pregnancy, the delays women may encounter, and the existence of any apparently complicated medical or social problems needing specialist attention. Particularly vulnerable are women from the lower social groups who tend to ask for help comparatively late in pregnancy. They are the least likely to be able to afford private treatment, and the least able to manipulate the public services to meet their needs. Their treatment may be speedier if the agency to which they are referred is sent detailed information about their background, and attention is drawn to the urgency of the situation. Some assessment should also be made of a woman's likely reaction to treatment, and she should be prepared for this. Women vary in their resilience to brusqueness and their ability to communicate with professionals. These considerations may all affect choices about sources of help.

Techniques of induced abortion

There are many methods of terminating pregnancies but the ones briefly described below are the most commonly used. These should be explained to women, although it is common for them to be told nothing about their operations. Ignorance increases fears and fantasies and makes women less likely to return for post-operative after-care.

In the first trimester of pregnancy it is normal for vaginal methods to be used. These are dilatation and curettage (D and C) and vacuum aspiration. In both cases the neck of the womb is dilated. With D and C a general anaesthetic is given and the contents of the womb are removed by forceps and curette. Most gynaecologists prefer not to use D and C after the twelfth week of pregnancy as the operation then becomes more difficult. Dilatation and curettage is not confined to abortion; it may be used after childbirth or a miscarriage and in connection with various gynaecological complaints. A woman should usually stay at least overnight in hospital after a D and C, and some doctors prefer longer stays.

With vacuum aspiration the womb is emptied through a plastic or metal tube attached to a suction machine. If this procedure is used early in pregnancy, by the eighth week if possible and not beyond the twelfth week, only a thin plastic tube is needed involving minimal stretching of the cervix. In this case only a local and sometimes no anaesthetic is necessary. The risks to the patient are therefore greatly reduced and she can leave hospital more quickly. Vacuum aspiration has made out-patient abortion possible, requiring only a few hours' stay in a clinic or hospital.

Women having out-patient abortions should have the procedure fully explained to them. They should also not have to travel long distances after the operation and, to ensure adequate after-care, they should be in contact with their general practitioners.

'Menstrual aspiration' is a term used for a procedure similar to vacuum aspiration but involves evacuating the contents of the womb before pregnancy can be easily diagnosed, that is in the first six weeks after a woman's last menstrual period. For a woman who fears she may be pregnant and who has consulted her doctor promptly menstrual aspiration may prevent weeks of anxiety. On the other hand, if she is not pregnant this procedure will have been unnecessary and also tends to be more painful than when performed in early pregnancy (Lane Report, Section D, 1974; Hindell and Grahame, 1974). So far menstrual aspiration has been very little used by doctors in Britain.

The methods of abortion most often used during the second trimester of pregnancy are hysterotomy and the use of drugs and other substances to stimulate uterine contractions which ultimately cause the expulsion of the foetus.

Hysterotomy is an operation performed under a general anaesthetic. The foetus is removed through an incision in the abdomen and then in the uterus. The wound heals but leaves a scar and that part of the uterus tends to remain weaker, entailing some risks during any subsequent pregnancy. These facts make hysterotomy more suitable for older women who have completed their families. A woman is often given hysterotomy if she also wants to be sterilised, since it is relatively simple for these two procedures to be combined. However, their combination increases significantly the risks of complications. After hysterotomy women need to stay in hospital for about a week followed by a period of convalesence of about two to three weeks. All these factors, especially the inevitably greater risks of a surgical procedure, make many doctors unwilling to perform hysterotomies, except as a last resort, and usually only after the sixteenth week of pregnancy.

Abortion can be induced without surgery by the injection of prostaglandin drugs or hypertonic solutions. Although the techniques of using these substances are improving the whole procedure may last about twenty to thirty hours and involves what is, in effect, a miniature labour. It can thus be painful and distressing, although it is safer than a surgical operation. There is also risk, after the use of prostaglandins, that the foetus may show signs of life, which, although minimal and of short duration, can be extremely upsetting for the patient and her attendants. This risk is slight when a pregnancy of less than sixteen weeks is terminated. When these methods of abortion are used women need support both during and after the procedure.

The risks of therapeutic abortion

It is not easy to give a precise and accurate account of the risks involved in terminating a pregnancy. This is partly because these vary according to the method of abortion and the duration of pregnancy, and partly because, to be meaningful, the complications of therapeutic abortion should be compared with those of childbirth. A pregnant woman is either going to have a baby or an abortion; both involve some risk. Also to be borne in mind in the assessment of continuing risks are the social and emotional implications of continuing the pregnancy (Illsley and Hall, 1975). Although there have been several studies of complications immediately following abortion, these are not always comparable because of the differing definitions used. Research in this subject may also reflect the attitudes of the researchers towards abortion, with dangers being emphasised or minimised accordingly. Study of the long-term after-effects of abortion both physical and psychological is even more hazardous, largely because of difficulties of follow-up after a long period, and because it can be hard to distinguish the effects of abortion from those of other trauma.

This section can therefore give only general indications of the risks involved in therapeutic abortions. Women need to be aware of these but counsellors who are not medically qualified should advise women to discuss them in greater detail with their doctors because their state of health will have some bearing on the likelihood and type of possible complication. Volume 1 of the Lane Report contains a comprehensive survey of research on the after-effects of therapeutic abortion (1974).

Physical complications

The most important principle to bear in mind is that the earlier in pregnancy an abortion is performed, the safer it is. Complications increase markedly after the twelfth week of pregnancy and they are also more likely when surgical procedures are used.

As doctors become more skilful in performing abortions, so do the risks decrease. In 1972 the fatality rate following all legal terminations of pregnancy was six per 100,000. The rate is considerably lower for abortions performed by D and C, or by vacuum aspiration before the thirteenth week of pregnancy; in 1971 this was 3.4 per 100,000 operations. By contrast the rate of maternal mortality (following all childbirth or pregnancy) in 1972 was eighteen per 100,000 births. When sterilisation is combined with abortion the fatality risk is considerably greater, as much as ten times greater when this accompanies a vaginal operation.

The chief complications immediately following therapeutic abortion are infection (sepsis) and haemorrhage. In 1971 the Registrar General recorded that overall, sepsis occurred in three cases and haemorrhage in six cases out of every 100,000 abortions performed before the thirteenth week of pregnancy. Their incidence is approximately twice as high for later abortions. However, it is known that the Registrar General's records are an underestimate of the rate of complications and some individual researchers report a considerably higher proportion of complications. Overall rates also conceal variations associated with different methods and periods of gestation.

Although the findings of studies of complications immediately following abortion, and especially early abortion, are reasonably reassuring, there is still some concern about its longer-term effects. There have been suggestions that the risks of spontaneous abortion and premature labour in subsequent pregnancies are increased when women have had a previously induced abortion. Definite conclusions about these possible complications can only be reached with prospective studies which compare the obstetric history of two carefully matched groups of women, who have had, and who have not had, a therapeutic abortion. So far the evidence there is, is inconclusive and conflicting.

Implications for mental health

Studies suggest that serious mental illness following an abortion can be expected in about 2 to 6 per cent of cases. Where there is such marked emotional distress and instability it is common for this to have been present in some degree prior to the pregnancy. A therapeutic abortion appears to have little influence, for good or ill, upon the course of an existing serious mental illness.

A larger proportion of women, perhaps about one-fifth, suffer more or less transiently from feelings of guilt, regret, self-reproach and a sense of loss. Strong feelings of guilt or bereavement may precipitate depression and may also lead a woman to become pregnant again. It must be remembered that this sadness and emotional distress are usally accompanied by a great sense of relief that a disaster has been averted and that an unpleasant episode is drawing to an end. Unhappy reactions will be most apparent to those caring for a woman immediately after an abortion, and since they rarely have such subsequent contact with her, they may imagine that these continue for much longer than is usually the case. The emotional distress and resentment of those involved in abortion work may exacerbate the women's own reactions.

Painful though these feelings are they should not necessarily be considered as pathological. However relieved a woman may be to have an abortion, to many this represents a loss for which they will mourn. Some may feel guilty that they did not use contraception wisely. An unwanted pregnancy is usually a serious crisis during which a woman may have to reassess her relationships with those on whom she thought she could rely; she may call into question her own moral standards; she may wonder about her future as a mother. In these circumstances it is natural, and indeed healthy, to expect some sadness and depression.

Women's reactions to treatment

It is sometimes said that patients' views of medical care should not be taken too seriously; they may not be in a position to understand fully the reasons for a doctor's actions or, in their anxiety, they may misinterpret what is being said to them. This cannot be a reason for not trying to achieve better communication between patients and doctors. Some understanding of women's reactions to treatment, and of the problems of medical staff, may reduce the tensions so often found between those involved in termination of pregnancy.

Cartwright and Lucas (1974) found that the women studied had two main criticisms. First, many women, especially if single, had found it difficult to talk to doctors, particularly hospital gynaecologists. Communication tended to be brusque and superficial. They therefore felt they had been unable to explain their situations fully, and that this had been a potent cause of misunderstanding. This study showed that most women were well aware that medical staff often disliked work involving termination of pregnancy, and some had a sensitive understanding of why this should be so. Occasionally objections to abortion were made plain to women and more usually they acted as an invisible barrier between the patient and those caring for her, and thus were a constraint on open communications (Macintyre, 1976a).

There were frequent complaints of lack of sympathy and understanding, and of some doctors, about one-tenth, being positively unhelpful. Even doctors who had helped women obtain abortions seemed, at times, intent upon making them feel guilty about their predicament and subjected them to scoldings and sermons. Nevertheless, in spite of these complaints, the great majority of women felt that their doctors had helped them in some way. They were also pleasantly surprised by the kindness and sympathy of their nurses, whom they had generally expected to be hostile.

If these findings do not seem to reveal too bad a situation, it should be remembered that Cartwright only studied women who had been successful in obtaining an abortion. It is probable that those who did not succeed would be more critical. The women in Cartwright and Lucas's study also had low expectations of their treatment. For example, while two-thirds had not been told what their operation would involve, only a quarter of these said they expected more information.

The second major complaint concerned frequent, and sometimes very long, delays in obtaining an abortion. These delays compound women's inevitable anxiety and may also mean using the riskier abortion procedures necessary later in pregnancy.

Nearly 90 per cent of the women in this study saw a doctor before nine weeks had elapsed since their last menstrual periods, and almost half had done this before six weeks had elapsed. If these women had been seen quickly at hospital the safest abortion techniques could have been used in most cases. In fact there were many delays, both in general practitioner and hospital consultations, and before women were admitted to hospital. Some of these delays arose because pressure on clinics meant difficulties in obtaining appointments, but many others were caused by general practitioners diagnosing pregnancy in slow and inefficient ways. Frequently abortion was not discussed during the first consultation with a general practitioner, sometimes because the doctor's manner made women diffident about raising the subject. Precious time was therefore lost. The routine of hospital consultation was not set in motion, and women also had less time to face up to their situation and think about this with professional help.

Limited resources

All public medical services are under acute pressure, with serious shortages of staff and other resources. When the Abortion Act was passed no special provisions were made to cope with the number of patients who would be referred to the NHS; in any case these have probably been much greater than was originally anticipated. Although it is often said that a high rate of abortion does not bring any extra work because, without this, the women concerned would need to be cared for during pregnancy and delivery, in the short term it is not easy to transfer resources for one kind of work to another, especially if this transfer is not generally welcomed by staff. Their attitudes have an important influence on the level of service (chapter 5, pp. 99-105).

Nevertheless, taken as a whole, the NHS has absorbed the

abortion work it has undertaken reasonably efficiently without, as is commonly feared, causing greater delays for other gynaecology patients (Lane Report, 1974). This does not mean that all hospitals have been able to cope equally well, and it is clear that in some abortion work has put an impossible strain on their resources. Furthermore, whatever the facts of the situation, medical staff believe that this work cannot be undertaken without detriment to other patients. Women requesting abortions appear as 'the grit in the system', the people who prevent doctors and nurses getting on with their 'proper work'. It is recognised that adequate assessments of their circumstances need more time than is usually available in out-patient clinics. Women requesting an abortion are also usually upset and tense, and their anxieties may quickly spread to staff and to other patients. Ways of reducing these anxieties are discussed in chapter 7.

Contraception

Understanding contraceptive dynamics will require sophisticated theory including the psychology of women, the psychology of the family, the value of children to parents, theories of death and dimensions of responsibility, control and time perspective (Bardwick, 1973, p. 302).

(Our study) suggests the overriding importance of some ability to communicate feeling associated with sex and contraception and to have these views sympathetically considered by both partners, and to act willingly on understandings developed from such communication (Rainwater, 1960, p. 138).

With the exception of that small minority whose unwanted pregnancies have resulted from a failure of one of the most efficient contraceptives, all parents unhappy about a pregnancy are likely to need some help with contraception. Numerous studies (Rainwater, 1960; Lambert, 1971; Cartwright, 1970; Bone, 1973; Williams and Hindell, 1972 and Pearson, 1973) have shown that although most men and women practise some kind of contraception, the majority tend to use unreliable methods, or to use potentially efficient methods sporadically and carelessly.

There are many reasons for inefficient contraception and apparently simple explanations of the associated problems may be only a veil for more complicated, perhaps only half-understood, anxieties about sexuality and fertility and the relationships between men and women (Rainwater, 1960).

Discussion about contraception

The context of a counsellor's work must inevitably influence the role he or she expects to play. Those who work mainly with mature, educated, middle-class, married couples will be much more aware of individual commitment to contraception than are those whose main contact is with the immature and the thoughtless, and those whose experience of life has taught them to submit to fate rather than to attempt to control their destinies.

Nevertheless, it is mistaken to ascribe to apparently homogeneous groups certain attitudes towards contraception and sexuality. Bardwick (1973), McCance and Hall (1972) and Rains (1971) found considerable sexual confusion and unhappiness, which influenced contraceptive behaviour, among a group of students with relatively sophisticated knowledge of contraception and a commitment to sexual relationships. Similarly, Rainwater's studies and the achievements of domiciliary family planning services have shown that couples who have been careless and unsuccessful in controlling their fertility can eventually, perhaps in desperation, learn to do this effectively.

Couples who act irrationally or irresponsibly in their use or neglect of contraception may need much more than explanations of contraceptive methods, and help with access to them. It is often wrongly assumed that a request for contraceptive help, or the mere existence of an unplanned or unwanted pregnancy, implies an unqualified commitment to the future control of fertility. In fact, both half-hearted and firm intentions to avoid pregnancy can be undermined by emotional conflicts within the individual and between sexual partners. Without some awareness of these conflicts it is hard to give appropriate contraceptive advice, or for methods to be chosen to which the couple can have some real, rather than theoretical, commitment. The technically most effective contraceptive will be unreliable if ambivalence towards it means irregular or careless use.

Vital though straightforward information and practical help are, they are too often given without sufficient regard to peoples' feelings about their sexual relationships, their future and their image of themselves as men and women and as parents. Contraceptive help must be offered to men and women, 'in terms of *their* realities, *their* understandings, *their* anxieties and *their* values and goals instead of simply in terms of "professionals'" own technical training and middle class point of view' (Rainwater, 1960, p. 174).

In discovering whether a couple's prime need is for information about methods and sources of assistance, or whether they need help to think more clearly about what the control of fertility means to them within this wider context, it may be helpful to explore why, at this point, help is being sought, what they already know about contraception and what their attitudes are towards it.

It is sometimes said that such enquiries are an unwarranted intrusion. Those who know what help they want should be allowed to have it without further ado. This seems a sensible view when people are quite clear what they want and there is a fair chance they will be able to use contraception effectively. Judging by the extent of unsuccessful use these two conditions seem often to be absent.

Without an invitation to give one's own views it can also be difficult to admit to doubts about contraception to those who seem strongly committed to the control of fertility, and especially if contraceptive carelessness has resulted in difficulties for other people. Not everyone will want to help with the problems that may emerge in the course of such a discussion and further counselling must be offered and not imposed. No doubt it will often be refused. A distinction can, however, be made between this extra help and a resolve not to discuss contraception in such a narrow context that complex needs meet with only superficial help.

Initiating discussion

It is sometimes said that it is unnecessary, and even unethical, for counsellors to initiate discussion about contraception, and that to do so may lead to many misunderstandings. However, Bone found that over a third of the women she studied (27 per cent of the middle-class and 41 per cent of working-class women) wanted to know more about contraception. Cartwright's (1970) studies also showed that two-thirds of those mothers who had not wanted their most recent pregnancy were attempting to control their fertility at the time they became pregnant. Marriage certainly did not mean instant sophistication in contraceptive practice and most of the people she studied thought that the subject of contraception should be raised by professional people. Couples are frequently too embarrassed to ask directly for contraceptive help and their oblique requests may well be ignored. This may partly account for the fact that 60 per cent of first births to teenage wives appear to be unintended. And since couples' intentions about family size are neither firm nor static and many are very uncertain whether they want another baby, they may welcome an invitation to discuss contraception (Cartwright, 1976).

Discussion of side effects

There is some evidence that people who have been informed of the potential problems and side effects of different contraceptives may experience them more frequently than those not given this information. On the other hand, if left in ignorance, at the first hint of difficulty men and women may become easily discouraged from continuing to use a particular contraceptive. Apart from these pragmatic considerations, people have a right to know something about the possible implications of different methods of contraception. Their reaction to this information will depend very much on how it is imparted. If the side effects of a particular method are rare or slight, it is foolish to preface a description of it with a long account of its potential problems. Difficulties also need to be set in their proper context. Are they likely to be greater or less than those arising from other contraceptives? And, most important, does the discomfort and nuisance of contraception outweigh the disadvantages of pregnancy for any particular couple?

It is unrealistic to expect no problems. According to the contraceptive methods used there may be physiological changes and some effect on physical sensation. Most contraceptives demand discipline and foresight and they may also prompt complex emotional responses. These reactions are more likely to be tolerated if ambivalence towards contraception is accepted as normal. If led to believe, erroneously, that there are no disadvantages to contraception, people may exaggerate any problems they experience and turn away from those who were not entirely honest in the help they gave.

Problems of access

Apart from the disadvantages associated with individual methods, to be discussed later, several studies have cited practical difficulties as the most important obstacles to successful contraception. There is no method of distributing contraceptive advice and supplies which meets everyone's needs. Clinics may be difficult to reach and held at inconvenient hours. If their sole aim is to give contraceptive help some find them embarrassing and off-putting. On the other hand, women may find it hard to approach people they already know for contraceptive help, thus excluding their general practitioners. Many unmarried people fear they will meet implied or actual moral opprobrium, and some do not think contraceptive help is given to single people. The young often find doctors and other professionals unsympathetic or unapproachable. In spite of the fact that contraceptive advice and supplies are now free to everyone from the National Health Service some think that the cost of contraception will be beyond their means. And no one likes to admit to ignorance which a request for help may imply.

That there are many inadequacies in contraceptive services is beyond doubt. Studies tend to focus on these, partly because they are relatively easy to study. It is then sometimes said either that improvements in services will resolve most, if not all, problems, or, that in spite of their shortcomings, services are within the reach of anyone with some persistence, and that failure to use them only highlights irresponsibility. While each of these conclusions may have some validity, taken on their own they ignore many of the more complex reactions to sexuality and the control of fertility. After all, Cartwright (1970) found that nearly a third of the mothers in her study disapproved of contraception. Less than half of these women were Catholics and there were many reasons for disapproval other than religious ones.

Reactions to sexuality

Efficient use of contraception depends very much on an individual's self-confidence, acceptance of his or her sexuality, and happy sexual and emotional relationships. Cartwright (1976) found that those couples who discuss contraception use it more effectively and tend to have smaller families than those who do not. One of Rainwater's most striking findings is that the married couples who were most satisfied with their sexual relationship were also those who practised contraception most effectively, partly because this satisfaction was associated with willingness to accept female methods. Those who are embarrassed, disgusted or frightened by their involvement in sexual relationships often find it difficult to ask for contraceptive help and will probably not be able easily to discuss contraception with anyone. Indeed, unmarried couples may not have acknowledged to themselves, or to each other, the sexual aspects of their relationship. Sexual intercourse can sometimes be an attempt to deeper communication rather than a result of this. It is of interest here to note Main's (1971) conclusion that the sexual lives of many of the women and girls who asked for abortion had been 'joyless, episodic and effortful with little of the confident anticipation that leads to unabashed and deliberate contraception. They all knew about contraceptives but the most immature were unable to think of themselves as sexual women who might use contraceptives' (p. 56).

This lack of self-confidence and enjoyment may be relatively superficial, arising largely from a person's inexperience, or it may be a legacy of parental embarrassment in discussing sexuality. More rarely it can be deeply rooted in an individual's personality, connected perhaps with an insecure childhood or unhappy relationships with parents. Quite frequently it can be both the cause and the product of marital unhappiness where a wife, perhaps in response to her husband's aggressive and self-absorbed sexual demands, rejects these wherever possible or submits to them with varying degrees of hostility (Rainwater, 1960).

Contraceptive practice can also reflect feelings about male and female roles in sexual relationships. Although there has been a long tradition in some family planning work that a woman's fertility ought to be under her own control, not least because the technically most efficient means of contraception are those used by women, it is now increasingly realised that it is difficult for women, particularly at certain stages in their lives, to take the contraceptive initiative. This implies a commitment to sexuality or to a relationship for which a woman may feel unprepared (chapter 4). Even when they accept this commitment women may still resent the fact that most men expect women to shoulder the whole responsibility for preventing pregnancy. It is not uncommon to find women, and especially those who derive little pleasure from sexual relationships, complaining that it is unfair that they should have the bother, embarrassment and possible discomfort of using contraception.

Fertility and parenthood

Many people who give contraceptive help, in their immediate response to an individual's desire to prevent pregnancy at a particular point in time, may fail to take into account that person's views and feelings about reproduction. They may think this would be an impertinence, that what has happened or will happen is an irrelevance, or they may simply be too busy to give more than immediate practical help. They may also wrongly assume that all women share the same reproductive instincts (Macintyre, 1976b). And yet an individual's feelings about parenthood must crucially affect contraceptive practice.

Most people's wishes and plans for parenthood are complex. The majority of couples desire at some stage to have more children than they actually have (Woolf, 1971: Rainwater, 1960). Economic and practical considerations, and perhaps fashion, make them change their mind. And yet for some there lingers on a concept of their ideal family size, or a picture of a good and unselfish woman as one who has several children. Despite their recognition of the practical difficulties in increasing their families, or their partner's opposition to this, they may hope for, or even contrive, an 'accidental' pregnancy. These hopes may partly account for an individual's commitment to an unreliable form of contraception or misuse of a reliable one.

Children are conceived, in spite of the practical and emotional difficulties this may mean, to deepen a relationship or to secure a faltering one. Some women admit that even though they realise a pregnancy would not prevent the break-up of a relationship the baby will be a precious reminder, almost a legacy, of someone they loved.

People will not usually admit to such apparently irrational, even irresponsible, states of mind. Their feelings about reproduction and about children, and the possible relationship of these to their use of contraception, will emerge only if they are given the opportunity to talk more widely than about their immediate need for contraception. Indeed, contraceptive counselling might well be more effective and helpful if it was seen more as counselling in relation to parenthood.

It is instructive here to observe how often men and women are angered by what they regard as the assumptions of those giving contraceptive help. Recently married women, who wish only to delay having children for a short time, may complain of the anti-masculine atmosphere of some family planning clinics, amounting almost, it seems to them, to a conspiracy against having children. This is the impression which, although quite unintended, may be gained by someone who has had little experience of contraception, who is given no chance to talk about parenthood, her plans or anxieties and who is told only about how to prevent birth.

Couples who do not ever intend to have children are equally infuriated by assumptions that this is only a temporary aberration, or worse still, by the implied criticism, still prevalent in a strongly natalist culture, that this represents either selfishness, or immaturity, or both (Peck, 1973).

Motivation for having children varies from culture to culture, and reasons may seem extraordinary, inappropriate, irresponsible or compelling according to an individual's cultural background and upbringing. Depending on a country's economy and arrangements for welfare and the relationship these have to family organisation, a large number of children may be seen as an economic liability, or as an eventual asset. For some the birth of children may bring prestige and complete recognition of their adult status, a confirmation of their fertility and potency. For religious or other reasons children may be seen as legitimising sexual relations; and there are certainly some women for whom pregnancy and childbirth are times when they feel most valued and worthwhile.

Having a family provides opportunites for parents to test their creative as well as their procreative powers; to some extent their children are an extension of themselves, an opportunity for vicarious achievement. They are also a source of fun and interest, the givers and receivers of love and affection.

To have or not to have children is one of the most important decisions men and women ever make, and it is usually a decision taken alone, perhaps because of the fear that discussion implies interference or even control over an aspect of an individual's life where he or she should have complete freedom. But people are not free when they cannot examine thoughtfully their own reactions to the highly emotional subjects of procreation and parenthood, or when they feel overwhelmed by pressures enjoining them to have, or not to have, children. They need to think about their own needs and aspirations and the best ways of achieving a fit between these and the circumstances in which they live.

This more wide-ranging counselling is not appropriate with every request for contraceptive help but it may certainly be relevant when an individual first asks for help, or when the practice of contraception seems to be sporadic or possibly when there is a request for a change of method, particularly if it seems this involves a change to a potentially less effective contraceptive. The aim should not be to ask intrusive questions, which are impertinent because they are not relevant, nor to press for a long discussion of an individual's sexual development and reproductive intentions, but to give an individual the chance to talk about the anxieties which so frequently surround sex and contraception.

Although it may help to explain why these discussions can be relevant to contraceptive practice, most counsellors find that people need little prompting to discuss matters of such great concern which are so frequently neglected. It is also more likely that contraception will be accepted if its positive role is emphasised, for example in enabling a higher standard of living, or more relaxed family life, rather than exhorting its adoption to prevent such disasters as acute poverty.

Attitudes towards the future

> Implicit in every plan is a belief in a more or less stable world: if one cannot assume a stable, predictable world it is very difficult to plan, since one cannot confidently imagine the conditions being planned for (Rainwater, 1960, p. 51).

Although men and women increasingly expect to have some control over their destinies and not to be mere victims of fate or natural forces, there remain large numbers of people whose experience of life has taught them that if is more realistic to attempt only minimal interference with the many constraints on their self-fulfilment. Indeed there are some whose inadequate education or whose wish to defend themselves from disappointments limits their awareness of these constraints. For such people, who are often the poorest members of the working class, planning and the implied long-term view of life are pointless and perhaps wrong, even if their day-to-day struggle to survive did not make them impossible. As Rainwater points out:

> The lack of effective contraception so common in this group is not due simply to ignorance or misunderstanding; it is embodied in particular personalities, world views and ways of life which have consistency and stability and which do not readily admit to such foreign elements as conscious planning and emotion laden contraceptive practices (pp. 167-8).

These assumptions frequently underlie the behaviour of that small minority who do nothing at all to prevent conception or who, after more pregnancies than they wanted, turn late and desperately to contraception.

Methods of contraception

There are many different methods of contraception some of which, if used efficiently, can give almost certain protection against pregnancy. But since there is no one perfect contraceptive, suitable for any individual at any stage in his or her reproductive life, simple to use and completely effective, with no unpleasant or dangerous side effects, individuals need help in choosing a method which will be best for them at that particular point in their lives. It is likely, therefore, that several different contraceptives will be used during a person's reproductive life, which will never be less than thirty years and for men is considerably longer.

It is generally agreed that the most effective contraceptive is not necessarily the one which is technically the most efficient, but the one an individual feels happiest in using. It is tempting, but often futile, for professionals to assume that they know best and to advocate medical methods of contraception which, although they may be the most effective, are unacceptable to the individuals concerned, not least because of their reluctance to ask for the help of professionals. In this respect the medical appropriation of contraception may present dangers and difficulties. Indeed, Cartwright (1976) suggests that propaganda against such methods as withdrawal and the safe period could be successful in discouraging people from using these methods without being successful in encouraging them to use other more effective methods.

Attitudes towards any particular method will depend partly on all the matters which have been discussed in the previous section, and partly on the nature and extent of a person's sexual relations. An individual who has sexual intercourse infrequently may not think it worth while using a contraceptive with long-lasting effects. The relationship between reproductive physiology and contraception also needs to be understood. Without this knowledge contraceptives may be rejected as unreliable.

There are many textbooks and booklets which discuss the technical aspects of contraception (Peel and Potts, 1969; Kleinmann, 1971). The intention here is to concentrate more on the relationship between contraceptive practice and an individual's life style, personality and aspirations.

Methods requiring deliberate action on each occasion of sexual intercourse: condom, withdrawal, diaphragm (cap), spermicides

With the important exception of the diaphragm, or the use of spermicides, these methods have to be the responsibility of the man. They may therefore be attractive to women who feel that men should take both the sexual and contraceptive initiative. This potential advantage has the accompanying disadvantage that women lose control over preventing pregnancy. If they are to feel safe from unwanted pregnancy they must have confidence in their partners' commitment to contraception.

These methods also have the advantage for couples who for various reasons, including possibly the sporadic nature of their sexual relations, do not wish to use contraceptives which provide continuous protection. It is, for example, unusual for a sexually inexperienced teenage girl who is unsure whether she will sleep with her boyfriend, and if so when, to take the pill in anticipation of this event. The most convenient and reliable method of contraception for young people in these circumstances is the condom. The pill is usually used only after a steady relationship has been established.

With the exception of the diaphragm, these contraceptive methods do not involve the ministrations of doctors or other professionals. They are usually easily obtainable and simple to use.

The condom (sheath or french letter) Condoms are most usually made of thin but strong lubricated latex and are designed to be fitted over the erect penis. There is usually a small teat at the end to hold the ejaculated fluid. After intercourse the condom is easily removed and thrown away. This is the contraceptive most widely used by married people and probably also by the unmarried. Bone (1973) found about three-quarters of married couples had at some time used condoms and about one-third were doing so at the time of her study. Although over 80 per cent of these were satisfied in some degree with the condom, less than half were completely satisfied with it.

Condoms are usually thought to be one of the safest methods of contraception, particularly if used in conjunction with spermicides. They also have the great advantage of being relatively cheap (about 5p each). Medical prescriptions are not needed for them and they can be obtained from clinics, chemists, slot machines, barbers' shops and by mail order. In addition, condoms provide some protection against sexually transmitted diseases. This fact, combined with the possible association of the use of condoms and illicit sexual relationships, may convey the impression that using them is disreputable, and therefore inappropriate for married couples.

The disadvantages of condoms are that some people find fitting them a nuisance which interferes with love-making and that using a condom can make intercourse less pleasurable for the man. Some also regard the tangible and physical barrier between the man and the woman unacceptable, while for others, who dislike the idea of contact between male and female genitals, or who feel more confident if the sperm never enters the vagina, this barrier is one of the attractions of condoms. A few couples also find condoms painful although this can usually be avoided by using a lubricating jelly. There may be anxieties that the condom may come off, split or have holes in it. Whilst all these things can happen they are most uncommon. Nevertheless, ideally spermicides should be used in conjunction with condoms to ensure protection.

Spermicides These may be obtained in the form of jellies, pessaries, creams or aerosol foams and are most usually used in association with condoms or the diaphragm. They can be obtained from family planning clinics and chemists without prescription. They must be inserted, usually with a special applicator, into the vagina a few minutes before sexual intercourse. They act by killing the sperm before these can fertilise the ova. Spermicides on their own are used only by a small minority of couples and are not a particularly safe method of contraception. Their advantages are that they are easy to use and virtually undetectable during love-making. On the other hand many couples find them messy and unaesthetic and have little confidence in them.

Diaphragm or 'dutch cap' These are made of rubber or plastic; usually they are round and dome shaped and held in this form by an outer ring containing a spring. The diaphragm is inserted by the woman into her vagina before sexual intercourse so that it covers the neck of the womb, therefore forming a barrier against sperm. The diaphragm should not be removed until at least six hours after love-making. If diaphragms are correctly fitted and used with spermicides they are one of the most reliable methods of contraception. Diaphragms are made in different sizes and have to be fitted by a doctor or specially trained nurse; a check-up is necessary at least once a year to ensure that the diaphragm is still the correct size for the woman. Women also have to be taught how to use them. This requires some basic knowledge of the female reproductive system and a woman's willingness to touch her genital area, including her vagina, and an ability to feel for the tip of the cervix to make sure the cap is in place. Bone found that about a fifth of married couples, most commonly from the middle classes, had used the diaphragm at some stage and although the great majority were satisfied with it in some degree, only about 40 per cent were completely satisfied.

For women who wish to be completely in charge of controlling their own fertility the diaphragm is one appropriate method. It has the advantage of being virtually undetectable during love-making and, if it is inserted regularly by a woman before every occasion she thinks she might have sexual intercourse, and ideally as part of the routine of going to bed, it need not interfere with spontaneity. However, this kind of commitment and preparedness is unusual and couples who rely on the diaphragm may often have to break off love-making for it to be inserted. This inconvenience means that couples may be strongly tempted to take risks.

Theoretically diaphragms can be useful for women who do not expect to have sexual intercourse very frequently; however, to avoid being without the diaphragm when they make love these women will have to be willing to admit to themselves the possibility that love-making will occur, even though they think it unlikely. For both the married and the unmarried this has both the advantage and the disadvantage of implying that the woman can be the initiator of sexual relations or is prepared for these before having been wooed and won.

A further disadvantage to the diaphragm is the anxieties felt by some women about having an object inside their bodies, and their belief that it can become dislodged and be ineffective or actually harmful. Some also find diaphragms messy to use and clean and fear they will be difficult to remove. However, for those couples who are strongly motivated to use the diaphragm, possibly because they fear the side effects of other reliable contraceptives, and who are able to plan ahead and incorporate its use into the rhythm of their sexual relationships, it can be an effective contraceptive.

Withdrawal or coitus interruptus, 'being careful' The oldest and still one of the most widely used methods of contraception is coitus interruptus where the man withdraws his penis from the woman's vagina before ejaculation. Bone found that nearly 40 per cent of married couples had at one stage relied on withdrawal and that it was more commonly used by the working class than the middle class. Surprisingly, given its obvious disadvantages, a substantial proportion of women whose partners used this form of contraception said they were completely satisfied with it. Other research suggests that most men are emphatic in their rejection of withdrawal as a desirable method of contraception (Rainwater, 1960).

The main advantages of coitus interruptus are that it does not require the couple to make any advance preparation, does not cost anything, does not require any professional consultation and has no medical side effects. On the other hand, if it is to be at all reliable it demands considerable awareness and self-control on the man's part to ensure that he withdraws soon enough. Sometimes he may think he has been successful whereas in fact some sperm have already been placed in the woman's vagina. It is also possible for men to deceive women by assuring them, wrongly, that they withdrew in time. In fact, although research has produced some contradictory estimates, coitus interruptus is generally thought to be one of the least reliable methods of contraception. In addition, withdrawal, and the anxiety it may mean for both partners, can prevent the woman from having an orgasm, and for some, coitus interruptus makes love-making unnatural and incomplete. The anxiety it may provoke is said sometimes to cause tension and frigidity.

As with all contraceptives, withdrawal is better than nothing, but it is certainly wise to discuss with couples using this method their reasons for doing so and their attitudes to more reliable and less disruptive kinds of contraception. Nevertheless, the extent to which coitus interruptus is used is a testimony to its acceptability, and for some couples it seems to become a normal part of love-making.

Methods not requiring deliberate action on each occasion of sexual intercourse: the pill, the intra-uterine devices (IUD), sterilisation

The most obvious advantages of these methods of contraception are their reliability and the fact that they allow for spontaneity in love-making. Their greatest disadvantages are their real, imagined or feared side effects, and the medical intervention they require. It is also said by some researchers that the reliability of these methods, and the fact that women are constantly able to have intercourse without fear of pregnancy, can mean problems for those who derive little pleasure from intercourse. Use of these methods means women cannot deter their partners by fear of pregnancy. Moreover, these contraceptives may imply an apparent commitment to sexual relations far greater than is actually the case, and this may increase unwelcome sexual demands. It is said that some women find a way out of this dilemma by emphasising the possible unpleasant side effects of the pill and IUD which leave them less able and willing to have intercourse.

These methods of contraception may, therefore, lead people to confront, perhaps for the first time, their sexual difficulties, and these problems are some of the hardest to acknowledge. These possibilities, and they are only possibilities, should be borne in mind by counsellors meeting men and women who, apparently for irrational reasons, are reluctant to use the safest forms of contraception, who abandon them without apparently good reasons, or who complain of side effects which seem to be exaggerated.

The pill Very briefly and simply the pill acts as a contraceptive by increasing the hormones in the woman's body which control the ovaries, thus preventing ovulation. The pill also has a number of other effects which make it difficult for the sperm to pass through the cervix and which reduce the ability of the uterus to accept the egg, even if fertilisation takes place. There are various different types of pill and in recent years their hormonal content has been decreased to reduce the side effects experienced by some women. To be completely effective a pill has to be taken every day, with a short break of five to seven days around the time of a woman's menstrual period. If used in accordance with the instructions for each type of pill it is the most reliable contraceptive available, its failure rate being reported as minute or non-existent. However, some routine and commitment is required for women to take the pill with unfailing regularity, and particularly with pills of low hormonal content, pregnancy may occur if they are not taken within twelve to twenty-four hours of the usual time. After condoms the pill is the most commonly used contraceptive, and nearly 70 per cent of users are said to be completely satisfied with it. The pill has to be prescribed by a doctor and women taking it need regular medical check-ups.

The convenience of the pill and its effectiveness make it an attractive method of contraception, and considerable efforts have been made by family planning organisations and doctors to promote its use. It has, however, several potential disadvantages, some of which appear to have been exaggerated, but which can be potent sources of anxiety and a deterrent to use.

The most serious criticism of the pill is that it increases the risk of thrombosis and pulmonary embolism, particularly if it is taken by women over the age of thirty-five. A great deal of research has been done on this subject for about ten years. This shows that although the pill increases these risks, if it is taken by women with no history of thrombosis, heart disease or certain blood disorders, it only does so very slightly, especially if the pill used contains little oestrogen. Regular medical check-ups also decrease these risks. Peel and Potts (1969) report that the overall mortality attributable to oral contraception is 2.2 per 100,000 in the twenty to thirty-four age group and 4.5 in the thirty-five to forty-four age group.

Any discussion of the possibly serious complications of the pill, although obviously necessary, may encourage people to focus on its disadvantages rather than on its greater advantages. It is as well, therefore, to bear in mind the fact that the risks of death from cigarette smoking, for example, are considerably higher than those from taking the pill. Sadly, these are greeted with far greater equanimity than the much smaller risks associated with the pill.

Less seriously the pill can cause weight gain, nausea, headache, breast tenderness, depression and break-through bleeding. There are, however, many other reasons for such conditions and without knowing how often they are experienced by women not taking the pill, it is difficult to calculate their significance. It is also possible that some women wrongly attribute various symptoms to the pill, perhaps quite sincerely, or perhaps as a mask for other anxieties they may have about using it.

The pill can also produce some beneficial side effects, such as the reduction or elimination of period pains and premenstrual tension; the amount or duration of menstrual bleeding is also often reduced. There are, however, some women who are distressed by these changes in menstruation, especially if they are not explained to them.

Discussion about the side effects and safety of the pill can be heated and irrational, and women have been berated both for their complaints and their equanimity in exposing themselves to alleged risks. Risks and side effects need to be acknowledged: their infrequency made clear; and they need to be compared with the risks of pregnancy and the side effects of other types of contraception. Apart from understanding these matters in general terms, the most important thing for a woman to know, with her doctor's help, is whether, in the light of her previous medical history, she has a greater or less chance of experiencing the pill's possible side effects. While it is important to allay women's unfounded fears that the pill is a serious danger to health, it is often unhelpful to ignore the fact that the pill does induce physiological changes. Most women taking the pill are likely to be aware of these. They will be less anxious if they are prepared for them and probably helped if their complaints of minor side effects are accepted as a part of the nuisance that the practice of contraception can mean. Ambivalence is the normal accompaniment of the mature weighing of the advantages and disadvantages of a method of contraception. It does not mean that someone is on the verge of abandoning it. Ignoring or denying complaints may make them much harder to tolerate.

Apart from these physiological side effects the pill can exacerbate emotional problems. These are not well understood and often ignored. The difficulties may be particularly great for unmarried girls whose sexual relations are, for various reasons, unsatisfactory. Bardwick (1973) found, in an admittedly limited sample of American college girls, a much greater degree of sexual anxiety and disappointment than had been expected given the professedly liberal and liberated attitudes towards sexual relationships. For many of these girls self-esteem was associated with a successful relationship with a boyfriend. They were also usually expected, and indeed most wanted, to take the contraceptive initiative. However, this could imply a premature commitment to sexual relationships and, for some at least, this meant undue importance being attached to the sexual aspects of their relationships with their boyfriends, from whom they were mainly seeking affection and security. Although some women believed that by removing the fear of pregnancy their ability to enjoy intercourse would be increased, for others their responsibility for sexual decisions aroused moral anxieties and guilt. Taking the pill meant facing up to their sexual desires instead of assuming that these were only the result of being swept off their feet in the heat of the moment. In spite of the much acclaimed sexual revolution, sexual activity and contraception were threatening to a group of women who derived little pleasure from sexual intercourse, and who were afraid they had degraded themselves and would be abandoned. These problems were particularly acute for women with low self-esteem who had little independent identity.

In these circumstances complaints about the pill would not be adequately dealt with by ignoring the anxieties which can surround the sexual relationships of both the married and un-married. Nevertheless, it must not be assumed that side effects are usually psychosomatic and therefore do not need to be taken seriously. Some women do experience disturbing and chronic symptoms, unrelated to their emotional state, which may necessitate changing to another method of contraception. And even if side effects do seem psychosomatic, they are still unpleasant and demand careful attention. They may be reduced by counselling but if they are not, another type of contraceptive may well be indicated.

Intra-uterine devices (IUD), the 'coil' These are plastic or metal objects in a variety of shapes and sizes which, when placed in the womb, prevent conception. IUDs have threads attached to them which pass through the cervix into the vagina to assist their removal. They are most suitable for women who have already had a baby but can be used by nulliparous women although they are then more difficult to insert.

There is some uncertainty about the exact way in which IUDs work. It seems most likely that they cause white cells to leave the blood vessels in the lining of the womb and to pass into the cavity where they can destroy the sperm on their way through the uterus to the uterine tubes where fertilisation takes place. They may also destroy the fertilised egg before it attaches itself to the wall of the uterus. There is thus some possibility that IUDs might be seen as abortifacients, although many biologists and theologians define conception as taking place only after the egg attaches itself to the wall of the womb.

There is a large variety of IUDs. It is important to explain how small they are, i.e. between one and three inches long and about one and a half inches wide. Ideally they should be shown to women who often imagine that they are very much larger and are anxious about having such an object inside them.

IUDs have to be inserted and removed through the cervix by doctors or specially trained nurses. Insertion usually causes little pain or discomfort although occasionally it can be very painful and require an anaesthetic. IUDs are sometimes inserted immediately after a pregnancy has been terminated or after a woman has given birth.

IUDs are at present used by only a small proportion of women, perhaps some 6 per cent, of whom the great majority are completely satisfied. After the pill, when it is taken correctly, IUDs are the most effective method of contraception. Very occasionally, however, uterine or tubal pregnancy does occur with the IUD in place and this may increase the risk of spontaneous abortion.

IUDs have the great advantage of not requiring any further action on the woman's part, apart from having a medical check-up shortly after insertion, and then perhaps only once a year. They also have the advantage and disadvantage, depending on a couples' attitudes, of making completely spontaneous love-making possible without fear of pregnancy. IUDs are also entirely within the woman's control, demanding only one firm decision that she wishes to be prepared for sexual intercourse. A similar decision has to be made if pregnancy is desired; with IUDs couples cannot hope for 'accidents'.

The disadvantages of IUDs are that they can cause heavy menstrual periods and some discomfort, although usually only for the first few months after insertion. Very rarely they may perforate the wall of the womb or cause pelvic infection. IUDs may also be expelled naturally although this is very rare with some of the newer forms. In order to check if the IUD is still in place women can be taught to feel for the threads attached to it.

Given their relative advantages and effectiveness it is not clear why IUDs are used by such a small minority of women, especially since some researchers have reported considerable interest in this method of contraception (Cartwright, 1970). Possibly before the introduction of free services some people were deterred by its cost. The insertion procedure and various fantasies about the side effects may also raise anxieties. Moreover, since only a minority of general practitioners fit IUDs themselves, the pill has been the form of contraception most commonly suggested by doctors.

Sterilisation   Both men and women can be sterilised and although the effects of this operation are sometimes reversible, sterilisation should be regarded as causing permanent infertility. Sterilisation for women has been available for many years but male sterilisation (vasectomy) for only about a decade. For legal, moral and religious reasons many doctors were, in the past, reluctant to sterilise women who had not already had several children or who were still relatively young. However, medical practice has changed considerably in recent years and sterilisation is now much more common, with many doctors being willing to sterilise young women who have had several children, or older women with only one or two. There are similar liberal attitudes towards male sterilisation. It is now usual for doctors to believe that couples themselves, provided they have been given adequate information and counselling, are the best judges of their need for sterilisation.

Female sterilisation involves cutting or blocking the tubes which carry the eggs from the ovaries to the womb. This can be done either by a small abdominal operation or vaginally. Depending on the method of sterilisation a woman is likely to remain in hospital for between one and seven days.

Male sterilisation (vasectomy) is a simple operation which can be performed on an out-patient basis. A local anaesthetic is injected into the skin of the scrotum; the surgeon then cuts each vas deferens, the tubes through which the sperms pass, and ties the end. The operation is performed well clear of the testicles and their hormones are not affected. After vasectomy a man should notice no difference in sexual desire or performance although there have been some reports of psychological disturbance in a small minority of sterilised men. The most common complications of this operation are local infection and some pain or discomfort. These are only troublesome in a small minority of cases.

Sterilisation for women performed within the National Health Service is free, and surgeons performing this operation for social reasons now receive extra remuneration. Vasectomy may also be performed free but more usually costs about £25. There may be considerable waiting lists for the operation.

Some couples fear that sterilisation will have the effects of castration or reduce the man's virility. Women may think that female sterilisation, especially if it includes hysterectomy (i.e. the removal of the womb), will mean that all their sexual and reproductive organs, including the vagina, are taken away. It is therefore important to explain that female sterilisation does not involve, damage or affect the ovaries which produce the eggs and female hormones, and that male sterilisation does not affect the testicles which produce the sperm and male hormones. These operations only stop the transmission of the woman's eggs and the man's sperm. The woman's eggs disintegrate in the uterine tubes and are easily re-absorbed. Infertile male sperm are continually being re-absorbed and this process is only increased when the vas deferens are cut. There are many new developments in methods of sterilisation and a couple should be advised to discuss these with a doctor.

Bone found that in her study only a very small minority of women (4 per cent) had been sterilised, although, not surprisingly, in the case of those who had had more than four children this proportion increased to nearly 25 per cent. About another quarter had thought about sterilisation, and again this proportion increased dramatically with the size of the woman's family. Rather more than half the women said they would prefer their husbands to be sterilised, usually because they realised that this was a simpler operation. Only a minority thought their husbands would be against sterilisation, although this was more common among working-class couples.

There is some dispute about the emotional after affects of sterilisation and there have been few reliable studies of these. Obviously for those couples who are sure they want no more children, who dislike or are unsuccessful with other forms of contraception, and who have both agreed that sterilisation is the best course, this can mean an enormous reduction in anxiety and freer, more relaxed love-making. But severe regrets, depression, or anxiety may occur when a decision has been rushed, or when doubts and fantasies about sterilisation have not been fully discussed, either by the couple or with the doctor or other counsellor.

Peel and Potts (1969) report that between 2 and 5 per cent of men and women regret their sterilisation and a great majority describe improved health and happier marriages. There has been some speculation that this high rate of satisfaction is to some extent a defence against the irreversability of the operation. If something cannot be changed adaptation or resignation are better than regrets. There may also be a higher rate of dissatisfaction among those with some previous emotional disturbance or unresolved doubts about sterilisation. There are, for example, some people who may rationally be fully convinced that they should have no more children but who wish that this were not so, and who may privately hope that circumstances will change to allow this. There are also couples where one partner is less in favour of sterilisation than the other, although willing to agree to this with greater or less reluctance. These doubts may have a religious basis; sterilisation is officially not permitted by the Roman Catholic Church although numerous Catholic couples and doctors decide they cannot in conscience accept this teaching. Anxieties may also arise, perhaps because the nature of the operation has been misunderstood, or because of the assault on the body sterilisation is assumed to be. It may therefore seem the most unnatural method of contraception. In somewhat unstable marriages, or where one or other partner is extremely jealous or suspicious, there may be fears that sterilisation will encourage unfaithfulness, since there is no risk of pregnancy resulting from sexual intercourse.

When there seems to be some disagreement or instability between couples it is therefore wise for sterilisation to be considered with even greater care than normal. Its irreversibility and the fantasies which may be associated with it may make other forms of contraception more appropriate. Against this must be set the advantage that sterilisation is the most effective method of controlling fertility and that once performed it demands no further action on the part of the couple or the medical profession.

Occasionally a woman asking for an abortion may be told, or imagine she is being told, that she can only have this if she agrees to sterilisation. Although this may be said with good intentions to women whose circumstances may well make sterilisation desirable, it is a cruel form of blackmail which can leave the woman with many regrets and much resentment.

Sterilisation is still a somewhat emotional subject and although it is becoming a much more common method of contraception, men and women are often shocked when the possibility is raised 'out of the blue' and with no discussion of their previous contraceptive practice. It is not a decision to be made when someone is emotionally disturbed, as women may be immediately before or after an abortion, or childbirth. It needs to be discussed with considerable sensitivity, and usually on several occasions. Both partners should be involved in these discussions. There are advantages in seeing them together and separately. Both should give their consent to the operation.

At present this kind of counselling would seem appropriate for most people. However, it must be acknowledged that there is a growing number of women, some of whom have had no children, who believe they have the right and ability to make a decision about sterilisation on their own, early in their lives and without help, or, as they might interpret it, interference from doctors and other counsellors. These requests or demands for sterilisation may, but certainly do not have to be, evidence of emotional disturbance. Whether they will become common and what the long-term effects might be are not yet known.

The rhythm method – the safe period

This method of contraception does not fall neatly under either of the previous two main categories. It does not require deliberate contraceptive action on every occasion of sexual intercourse, nor is it a method which, once adopted, provides regular protection for a long period. Very simply, the safe period is that time before and after ovulation when a woman is less likely to conceive. The human egg is released from the ovary about fourteen days before the beginning of a menstrual period. If not fertilised it usually degenerates within two or three days, perhaps sooner. Sperm which reach the uterus or uterine tubes are probably capable of fertilising the egg for two to three days. In theory, therefore, if couples abstain from sexual intercourse for about seven days at the time of ovulation conception should not take place.

Calculating the safe period reliably is not easy and couples should seek professional advice about how to do this. Very briefly the woman has to record, preferably over a period of six to twelve months, the onset of menstruation and the length of her cycle. From this information it is possible to calculate the days when ovulation is likely to occur. This calculation may be extremely difficult, if not impossible, for women with irregular menstrual cycles, and couples may therefore have to resign themselves to the fact that they can only regard about half of the days of the menstrual cycle as being safe.

Alternatively, and more accurately, it is possible to calculate the period of ovulation by recording a woman's temperature which rises slightly when ovulation takes place. If this temperature rise is maintained for at least seventy-two hours, with no infection or illness to account for it, it is safe to say that ovulation has taken place at the beginning of the rise. If intercourse is avoided from the beginning of each menstrual cycle until seventy-two hours after the temperature rose, by which time the egg should no longer survive, then conception is highly unlikely in the rest of the cycle.

Some couples may use a combination of the calendar and the temperature method of calculating ovulation. If a woman has a regular menstrual cycle, and therefore expects to predict the time of ovulation with some accuracy, a prediction which can be confirmed by taking her temperature, it may be reasonably safe for her to have intercourse during the time between the beginning of her menstrual cycle and the expected time of ovulation. Unfortunately, the interval between the previous menstruation and ovulation, which is the period which needs to be predicted in order to use the rhythm method successfully, is often irregular.

Some researchers suggest that, if used properly, the safe period is an extremely effective method of contraception, but because of the difficulties of calculating the time of ovulation, and the self-control involved, reliance on the safe period does not usually prove to be a reliable method of preventing pregnancy. It is reported to have one of the highest failure rates of any contraception. Bone found that 13 per cent of couples had at some stage used the safe period and, perhaps surprisingly in view of its disadvantages, about 40 per cent of these were completely satisfied with it.

The safe period's disadvantages are the intelligence and skill required in calculating it, and the strain imposed by abstinence from intercourse for quite long periods each month, and its unreliability.

The advantage of using the safe period is that it requires no pills or artificial aids, with the possible exception of a thermometer. Some couples may therefore regard it as the most natural contraception. It is also the only method of controlling fertility officially permitted by the Roman Catholic Church which at various times has condemned other methods of contraception. This approval may be important for some Catholic couples who are more likely than non-Catholics to use the safe period. However, many Catholic bishops and priests, together with a very large number of the laity, do not agree with their Church's teaching on contraception and have chosen to follow their own consciences in this matter. Cartwright's and Bone's studies both showed that artificial methods are used almost as widely by Catholics in Britain as by non-Catholic couples. What is not clear is whether these Catholics who use contraception do so as early in marriage as non-Catholics and to what extent, in spite of the advice of many of their clergy that they should follow their consciences, they feel guilty about their behaviour. The varying degrees of liberality with which Catholic teaching is interpreted in different countries, and at different educational levels, will affect the answers to these questions.

It may well be appropriate when discussing contraception with Catholic couples to be sensitive to moral doubts or queries. For those couples who would be helped by having some religious sanction in their use of contraception it is usually possible in Britain, and in several other European countries, to refer them to a priest with liberal views.

Addresses of the headquarters of useful organisations

Welfare Benefits and Accommodation

Child Poverty Action Group (CPAG), 1 Macklin Street, London, WC2 5NH. Telephone no. 01 242 3225.

Citizens' Rights Office, 1 Macklin Street, London, WC2 5HN. Telephone no. 01 405 4517.

Gingerbread, 9 Poland Street, London W1V 3DG. Telephone no. 01 734 9014.

National Association of Housing Societies, 86 The Strand, London, WC2R 0EQ.

National Council for One Parent Families, 255 Kentish Town Road, London, NW5 2LX. Telephone no. 01 267 1361.

Shelter Housing Aid Centre, 189a Old Brompton Road, London, SW5 0AR. Telephone no. 01 373 7276.

Adoption

Association of British Adoption Agencies, 4 Southampton Row, London, W1CB 4AA. Telephone no. 01 242 8957.

Abortion

British Pregnancy Advisory Service (BPAS), Guildhall Buildings, Navigation Street, Birmingham, B2 BBT. Telephone no. 021 643 1461.

London Pregnancy Advisory Service, 40 Margaret Street, London, W1N 7SB. Telephone no. 01 409 0281.

Contraception

Family Planning Association, 27-35 Mortimer Street, London, W1. Telephone no. 01 636 7866.

Brook Advisory Centres, 233 Tottenham Court Road, London, W1P 98E. Telephone no. 01 323 1522.

seven

Aspects of counselling

The purpose of this last chapter is to discuss techniques and problems of counselling in relation to unwanted pregnancy, and to focus on particularly vulnerable groups. It is assumed that readers will be familiar with the basic objectives and methods of counselling; if not, Venables's (1971) short book and the rather longer ones by Wallis (1973) and Bessell (1971) provide good introductions. Bird (1973) also discusses briefly and helpfully the handling of day-to-day problems patients bring to their doctors.

What relevance do the most common elements of counselling, the expression and clarification of feelings, practical help and emotional support, have to men and women anxious about a pregnancy?

The clarification of feelings

The problems which surround unwanted pregnancy are emotive and controversial. It is common for the couples concerned to be overwhelmed by deep and confusing feelings, and seeing their interests as neglected or misunderstood, to be resentful and angry. Guilt, anxiety and embarrassment make if difficult for these problems to be discussed openly. Men and women are thus drained of emotional energy and at greater risk of making muddled decisions. Feeling deprived themselves they cannot give freely to others.

The first four chapters of this book explain how the very mixed experiences and emotions which accompany pregnancy and parenthood are an essential part of the human condition, and especially likely in a period of rapid social transition when new opportunities, new satisfactions and new discontents emerge. To acknowledge only parents' positive feelings about pregnancy increases their anxiety. Couples need to be reassured that questioning the implications of parenthood is natural and responsible. It is not a symptom of failure, nor should it be the object of social disapproval.

Mothers with young children are especially vulnerable to the conflicting pressures of contemporary society. Their well-being, and that of their dependants, will depend partly on the opportunities they have to control that part of their lives which can be controlled, and to plan what can be planned. These opportunities may well be missed if women are unclear about their feelings or unable to cope with the sense of drifting discontent, confusion or panic which can accompany pregnancy.

If counsellors believe that pregnancy and early motherhood can be an important stage in a woman's development they will welcome the opportunity of offering help at a time when it can be so well used. The opportunity for rapid change, for the reappraisal and resolution of older conflicts as a woman explores her identity as a mother, comes about because of her tendency in pregnancy and after delivery to be more than usually in touch with her feelings and memories of important influences on her (chapter 3). It is therefore usually unnecessary to probe deeply into a woman's past in order to understand her present. She is doing this work herself and all that she usually needs is help to relate what is so vivid to her anxieties about motherhood. A further advantage is that women at this stage in their lives appear to need, and to be able to make, speedy and helpful relationships with someone who is friendly, dependable and interested in them for their own sake, not just in their baby (Caplan, 1961; Kitzinger, 1962).

Counsellors need to be aware that both they, and the women they are trying to help, may be surprised and frightened by the swings of mood, the vividness of recall and the intensity of feeling, which seem to characterise pregnancy and early motherhood. Women should be helped to keep in touch with these feelings, to share those they are ashamed of, and to explore differing images of motherhood. The open expression of anxieties during pregnancy can help adjustment to maternity (Breen, 1975). The risks of neglecting unspoken conflicts are far greater than the risks of appearing to interfere.

The following case studies show how individuals given help to clarify their feelings were able to understand better the relationship between the inner world of fantasy and emotion and their behaviour.

A student and her boyfriend

Jill, a student with a long-standing relationship with her boyfriend, had visited a family planning clinic at various intervals and had been prescribed the pill. When, during a check-up, the doctor asked if she needed further supplies she was at first mystified by Jill's reply that she still had lots of pills; she had not been using them regularly and that she did not therefore need a check-up. She also blurted out that she thought she might be pregnant. In the course of discussion it emerged that Jill had no fears of the pill and had experienced no side effects, that her relationship with her boyfriend was happy and they planned to marry when they had completed their studies. A baby before then, said Jill, would be disastrous. What explanation could there possibly be for her apparently irrational behaviour? Jill seemed keen to discuss this further, and in two more meetings told the doctor that in spite of her happy relationship with her boyfriend and her apparently settled future, she felt deeply confused. She found her academic work rewarding but difficult. Although at times tempted to give it up, she feared that if she did so, settling for a life of domesticity or a less demanding job, would leave her dissatisfied.

Jill's mother, described as happily married and without a career, had apparently always been ambitious for her. She and Jill were very close and Jill was aware that her mother was both keen for her to succeed in her academic work, and to marry and have several children with whom she, as grandmother, would be actively involved. But Jill's mother, although she seemed to be pushing her in both directions, also appeared to see these two possible futures as mutually exclusive, and so, to some extent, did Jill. She had no experience within her own family of a combination of employment and motherhood and thought, realistically, that this would anyway be difficult until she had established herself in a career. Her boyfriend appeared open minded about which course she pursued. There was, Jill acknowledged, a strong part of her that wanted to give up her studies, particularly as the hurdle of the examinations drew nearer. If she became pregnant this indecision would be removed from her. She certainly would not contemplate an abortion; she and her boyfriend would marry and she would be content. But would she? It was this nagging doubt which had lured her to ask for help, albeit in an oblique way.

Jill, who was not in fact pregnant, talked for some time about her anxieties over her exams, her deep-rooted need to do well, and to please her mother, and her confusion about how this might be achieved. She also, guiltily at first, but then with relief, expressed some hostility towards her mother's apparently conflicting encouragement and towards her boyfriend's non-committal approach. Jill was encouraged to talk to him and also to her mother about her dilemma. She subsequently told her doctor that her boyfriend had been delighted to share this problem. He had previously felt that it was something she wanted to sort out on her own or with her mother. Jill had not felt able to have a proper talk with her mother about her confusion but said that with her boyfriend's support and her new understanding of the pressures on her she felt much more at peace with herself. She resumed taking the pill, decided to sit her examinations and pursue her career, at least for a few years. She recognised that she would probably always feel some tension between this and motherhood.

A middle-aged mother

Mrs Everett, thirty-nine with three adolescent children, had planned for a long time to open a small shop when her family needed her less. They were not well off but her husband had helped her raise a small loan and the shop was due to open in a few months. Then Mrs Everett found she was pregnant. She told her doctor she was horrified and deeply distressed about this. She could not face, at this stage in life, the care of another infant; she was longing for the independence of work; she already had heavy financial commitments. She must therefore have an abortion. She concluded all this outpouring with the remark: 'perhaps being a mother is all I'm good for.'

The doctor picked this up and Mrs Everett confessed that she was extremely nervous about her new venture. She had not worked since she was eighteen; she was totally inexperienced in business; she often lay awake worrying about the debt. And, she said tearfully, 'I do love babies. I am good at looking after them. I often wish the others were still small children.' When asked how it was she became pregnant, since she had been an efficient user of contraception, Mrs Everett said that recently she had not been using her cap because she thought it did not fit. She saw immediately how illogical this was and agreed with her doctor that, whatever her avowed intentions, her behaviour seemed to show she wanted two things: a return to motherhood and a more independent future. She was advised to think about this further and returned two weeks after to say that she and her husband had decided that she should have an abortion and then be sterilised. This was consistent with her long-term plans, and although the conception had shown how ambivalent she was about her future, she felt convinced for her own sake and for her family that she should pursue her original aim. 'I cannot always be a mother of infants. I have to establish a new life for myself. I believe I can do it.' For Mrs Everett these two weeks had been a time to reappraise herself and her family, to mourn for her past identity and to plan for her future.

Giving information

Giving information about such emotive matters as contraception, abortion and adoption, and the possible implications of illegitimacy, is a much more complex task than it may at first appear. Even though aware of their need for information, anxious people may not hear or be able to make use of what is said to them. One of the skills of counselling is recognising this anxiety and trying to alleviate it. This cannot be done by giving false reassurance. A woman who is unhappy about her pregnancy has much to worry about and anticipatory worry is a sign of health and an impetus to planning (Caplan, 1961). However, it is easy for anxious people to confuse fantasy and reality and they may need help to disentangle these. In these circumstances information may have to be repeated and discussed several times before it is digested and used effectively. In their anxiety men and women may well resort to previously discarded fantasies. Their counsellors need then to show them what is happening and to hold on to reality.

Imparting information is not a separate stage of counselling. It permeates the whole process and raises for counsellors questions about the initiatives they should take. It is relatively easy to provide information which has been requested, but how far should counsellors mention subjects which they think may be shocking, or at least rejected, almost out of hand? Should people be allowed to make grave decisions before they have carefully considered all the possible options? Are there not risks in putting ideas into people's heads, or of undermining their confidence by unpalatable truths?

It is unlikely that a couple has not at some stage contemplated all the various ways of coping with an unwanted pregnancy. They may, however, be embarrassed to admit this and briskly dismiss information about some of the options before them. The counsellor has then to decide whether it would be easier for these to be considered more fully when a person feels more at ease, or whether it is unrealistic to pursue the matter, either because of staunch opposition to it, or because of the unproductive distress such discussion might cause. This decision will depend partly on the counsellor's understanding of the meaning of the pregnancy to the couple, and whether this seems to be largely accidental or intended, if only in a half-conscious and confused way, to meet their needs. Decisions about the imparting of information may also be influenced by counsellors' own values, although it is good practice to assume that a couple will co-operate in an honest examination of all the alternatives before them. Such a discussion is both a sign of maturity and a step towards it.

It may be especially difficult to work with couples who seem emotionally flat and apathetic, apparently unconcerned about their dilemma but who, at the same time, appear to be asking to have something done for them. Cruel though it may seem to disturb their unruffled surface, a counsellor has a responsibility to discuss the options before them and the difficulties they are likely to face, whether or not the baby is born.

> The important point is to stress the real detail of what they will perceive. You do not have to go into all the painful possibilities of what they are not likely to perceive. The thing to do is to talk about the things you know they are likely to hear, and feel, and smell afterwards. It should not just be a nice story (Caplan, 1961, p. 56).

Counsellors have therefore to observe carefully reactions to information being given and, if they are unsure about whether it has been understood, to ask what has been heard. Anxieties about referral to other sources of help must also be watched for. It is never easy to ask for help, and especially hard when this will involve discussing apparently shameful or embarrassing subjects. Furthermore, anxious people tend quickly to become dependent on those who first help them in their crisis. Entrusting oneself to another person may be a wearisome or frightening prospect. This needs to be discussed and, as far as possible, detailed information given about the new source of assistance. It can be helpful for a counsellor to make the initial contact and to accompany someone on a first visit to an unfamiliar agency.

Practical help and emotional support

Caplan (1961, p. 56) has said that women faced with the inevitable anxieties of pregnancy 'should worry, in the presence of support, and in an atmosphere of hope'. What support can a counsellor give?

Not every woman anxious about her pregnancy needs practical help, although many do. Shortage of resources, the difficulties of mobilising help outside a counsellor's own agency, preoccupation with underlying pathology and sheer lack of imagination, too often dim this crucial awareness of material needs (Weir, 1970). Counselling those who are beset with the multitudes of problems which can accompany unwanted pregnancy must often be more than just sitting, listening and discussing. If the help needed is unlikely to be available, this should not be ignored. Awareness of the gap between needs and resources is the first step towards more adequate provision.

All counselling, whether or not it includes practical assistance, should provide some emotional support and there are many men and women whose greatest need is for this rather than any other help. Emotional support is an essential part of the clarification of feelings which was discussed earlier. It comes about when people feel that their counsellors are genuinely interested in them and care about them, that they understand, or are trying to understand them, and that they are not shocked or frightened by what they hear (Truax and Carkhuff, 1967). Helpful relationships offer much more than reassurance and the exchange of pleasantries; they are the context in which uncomfortable subjects can be examined and individuals can feel accepted in their entirety, their badness as well as their goodness.

These relationships may at times be very intense. In their crises and anxiety women faced with an unwanted pregnancy can become extremely dependent. This dependence is compounded by the power many counsellors possess, or are believed to possess. In such a situation individuals' behaviour may well be coloured by their memories of their own parents and other people who have greatly influenced them (Kitzinger, 1962). Here may lie the roots of apparently inappropriate fear, hostility or gratitude. Hard though it can be to tolerate these reactions, this can be an essential step in helping individuals to recognise and come to terms with earlier experiences which still cast their shadow on their behaviour.

The following case study illustrates these three aspects of counselling. It should be observed that while considerable sensitivity was required to understand this family's needs, the help given was relatively simple.

Mr and Mrs Floyd and Edward

Mrs Floyd was twenty-three and had been married for two years when she became pregnant. She and her husband had been using contraception and the pregnancy was quite unintended. Mr Floyd had a junior office job and was working and studying hard to gain promotion. The couple were not well off and Mrs Floyd had intended to continue working for some years as a secretary, partly to contribute to the family income and partly because she very much liked her work.

Mrs Floyd and her husband were dismayed to discover her pregnancy. They hoped for a miscarriage and wondered about an abortion, although Mr Floyd was uneasy about these possibilities. He thought that his wife would come to accept the baby and that despite financial difficulties, they would probably manage. Mrs Floyd was not so sanguine; she desperately wanted to be rid of the pregnancy, but on seeing her husband's reaction was frightened that if she pursued the idea of abortion he would think her callous and unfeminine. She dreaded giving up her job since she felt it gave her an identity and some importance. It was also a distraction during her husband's long working hours. In any case both Mr and Mrs Floyd thought that it would be unlikely that, given their circumstances, a request for an abortion would be granted. They both felt rather ashamed about their response to this pregnancy and thought they would be strongly criticised if it was known they wanted to end it. Nevertheless, in the vain hope that her real feelings would become apparent without having to state them explicitly, Mrs Floyd told her general practitioner that the pregnancy had not been planned and that the arrival of a baby would be difficult for her and her husband. She also said she wondered if she would have a miscarriage. Her doctor failed to respond to these cues and only remarked that many young couples faced similar difficulties, and that it was unlikely she would have a miscarriage.

Mrs Floyd remained anxious, tearful and depressed throughout her pregnancy. Her husband, who was preoccupied with his work, thought this was a more or less normal condition and Mrs Floyd did not feel able to discuss with him her continued dread of having a child. The conventional responses of delight and congratulations from parents, in-laws and friends confirmed Mrs Floyd's feelings that her response to her pregnancy was largely unnatural, and since it would not be understood or accepted, should be hidden as far as possible. As if she were trying to deny the existence of the pregnancy Mrs Floyd did not go to the relaxation or mothercraft classes provided by the hospital. She continued to work until the very last weeks of pregnancy and was greatly distressed when she finally left her job. She did not seriously consider working after the birth, partly because she assumed the practical difficulties would be insuperable, but largely because she felt that this would attract strong disapproval. She also thought she would be failing in her duty as a mother. Although Mrs Floyd's doctor was aware of her depression he responded by reassuring her that she would feel much better later in pregnancy, or if not then, after the baby was born. He said it was natural for her to feel somewhat lonely and worried at such a time. Mrs Floyd realised that the doctor was quite unaware of the origins of her misery, and her fear of criticism or reproach made it impossible to spell them out.

After her baby was born Mrs Floyd was not surprised when she did not experience the rush of maternal feelings which she had been promised by so many people. She was tearful and tired and felt no pleasure in caring for her son. She did not want to breast feed but agreed to do so under pressure from nurses. She quickly gave this up when her baby did not respond easily, and was dismayed to find that he also did not feed well from a bottle. Whenever possible she left the nurses to feed and bath Edward and she was reluctant to have him near her in the ward. She did not want to be discharged from hospital and complained of various minor ailments to delay this. Although this behaviour was noted by the medical staff as being somewhat unusual it was briskly put down to post-partum 'blues'. Again Mrs Floyd was cheerfully assured that most young mothers felt as she did some of the time, that she had a lovely baby and that she would cope very well as soon as she got home. In the face of such buoyant, if insensitive confidence and apparent total commitment to motherhood and young babies, Mrs Floyd did not dare admit her real feelings.

Not surprisingly Mrs Floyd did not manage well when she got home. Edward continued to be difficult to feed and was constantly fretful. Mrs Floyd felt exhausted and miserable at her failure to cope with his incessant demands and her resentment of this unwanted imposition. Now actually faced with the responsibility for Edward, Mrs Floyd felt even less able to admit openly that she did not want and did not love him. Her husband was worried by her failure to cope but assumed that things would become easier.

At her first visit Mrs Johns, the health visitor, was concerned by Mrs Floyd's apparent depression, tiredness and tight-lipped responses to questions about the baby. She noticed that, although Edward was in the same room, Mrs Floyd did not offer to show him to her nor did she make any movement towards him during a fairly lengthy discussion. She resolved to call again soon and suggested that Mrs Floyd contacted her if things continued to be difficult.

At her second visit it was apparent that the problems had worsened and Mrs Johns thought that Mrs Floyd seemed not only exhausted and depressed but very angry. This impression was confirmed when, in response to a gentle query as to why Mrs Floyd had not got in touch with Mrs Johns as she had suggested, Mrs Floyd burst out that she had not done so because nobody understood what she felt and what she was going through. Mrs Johns said that she thought Edward was a difficult baby and it was very depressing and unnerving to have all one's efforts at caring apparently rejected. As Mrs Floyd's response to this was a sullen silence Mrs Johns said that she thought Mrs Floyd must sometimes wish the baby was not there at all and she could get out of the house and do something interesting. At this Mrs Floyd suddenly blurted out that Edward was a hateful baby, she had never wanted him and she wished she had got rid of him. She then burst into tears and sobbed that everyone would think she was wicked and a failure. Mrs Johns did not attempt to stop her crying or cheer her up, but when she was calmer she remarked that it was not at all uncommon for women not to want babies, although it was often made very difficult for them to admit this. It was not always easy for those who had no children, or who worked in maternity hospitals, or who had always wanted their own children, to imagine the feelings of those women who did not want their babies. This prompted Mrs Floyd to explain her attempts to communicate her unhappiness to her doctors and her ploys in hospital to draw attention to her predicament. Mrs Johns then asked if she would like to explain why she had not wanted the pregnancy. When this was done Mrs Johns said she thought the reasons were perfectly understandable and sensible. She hoped Mrs Floyd would talk to her more about them on other visits.

Mrs Johns visited Mrs Floyd for some months and in the course of their discussions Mrs Floyd was able to look in greater depth at her panic at becoming pregnant and her distress at giving up work. Apart from all the practical problems this presented Mrs Floyd explained how she had dreaded having a life like her mother's, which had been totally dominated by the care of children. While she had encouraged Mrs Floyd to qualify as a secretary, she had always said that her main job in life would be caring for children. It had often been implied that only women with children were truly fulfilled, and that those who were committed to their work were in some ways unwomanly. Although Mrs Floyd did not agree rationally with these views she acknowledged she had been deeply affected by them. She had felt that she would be diminished as a person if she admitted to not wanting her child. She thought that everyone, including her husband, would see her as unfeminine and unnatural. Indeed, she felt this herself.

Given the opportunity to talk in this way, to see this stage of motherhood as only one phase in her life, to discuss more effective methods of contraception, and to look at the various possibilities of alternative care for Edward, Mrs Floyd's panic and misery seemed to decrease. Judging her relationship with her husband to be a basically good one, Mrs Johns encouraged her to discuss her difficulties with him. Supported by the fact that someone had taken her predicament seriously, and not been shocked by her reactions, Mrs Floyd did this and discovered that her husband too fully accepted her feelings. He had in fact suspected them but had feared his wife would be deeply hurt by these suspicions. Responding, no doubt, to the less tense atmosphere, Edward became a more contented baby and Mrs Floyd began to feel that, at least in practical terms, she could cope as a mother.

Although Mrs Floyd had been tempted to return to work as soon as possible she also thought that to do this might be a sign of her inadequacy as a mother. She was therefore much helped by Mrs Johns's comments that to be an apparently dutiful parent while not enjoying this could be very unsatisfactory for the whole family. Given the option of looking at different ways of fulfilling a maternal role, she felt she could relax while making up her mind. Eventually she decided to take in some work at home and when Edward was older she arranged, through the help of Mrs Johns, for him to go some afternoons a week to a child minder. This worked reasonably well and Mrs Floyd was greatly relieved to find that she could shape her life, at least partly, according to her own wishes.

Most interesting of all was Mrs Floyd's response to Edward. Reassured that it was neither a disaster nor peculiar for her not to have wanted Edward, or to feel able to love him at birth, she decided, in her own words, 'to get along with him and see how it goes'. After a few months she told Mrs Johns that she now could not imagine being without him, even though she could see some of the advantages of this. As Edward became more responsive she found herself, almost unawares, talking to him and playing with him and, she wrily admitted, 'actually quite enjoying it'. In this she was helped and supported by her husband, who was extremely fond and proud of Edward, and who now felt free to express his affection without fear of irritating his wife or making her feel guilty.

As Mrs Johns watched the bonds grow between Mrs Floyd and Edward she realised that Mrs Floyd would feel increasingly guilty about her initial response to him and would probably worry about its effect on their future relationship. She discussed this with Mrs Floyd who agreed that even now she felt she often did not treat Edward fairly. At times she would be depressed, impatient and unresponsive and then, feeling ashamed of this, she would over-indulge him. She was quick to blame herself for any of his difficulties. It helped her to discuss the problems this can mean for children, and to be reassured that parents who had always wanted their children could react in exactly the same way.

Mrs Johns also tried to help Mrs Floyd to accept herself as she was, and not to worry constantly about how she fitted in with conventional preconceptions of what women should be and do and feel. She needed to discover what sort of person she was, and wanted to be, and why. Mrs Floyd agreed that having Edward had made her and her husband sort out, perhaps too early for comfort, some basic questions about themselves. For example, she came to the conclusion that, in spite of her many abilities, she lacked self-confidence. This had received a serious blow when she could not cope with the baby, and although her now proven competence as a mother helped her, she realised that she would always be concerned about the opinions of others and conforming to their expectations. She would continue to need not only the interest and stimulus of work but the reassurance this gave her of her worth.

These problems left their scars. Mrs Floyd's relationship with Edward was more complicated than the one that developed with her second planned and wanted child, born four years later. She looked back on her first pregnancy and Edward's birth as the most unhappy time of her life and, in spite of reassurance and the passing of time, remained deeply sad about her early response to him. She was inclined to brood about herself and her worth as a mother and a wife. But she never again experienced the panic, confusion and resentment that overwhelmed her at Edward's birth. He became happily established in the family, and although his parents saw that he had certain difficulties, they understood these and felt reasonably able to cope. The relationship between Mr and Mrs Floyd grew stronger as they found it easier to share their thoughts and feelings.

Undoubtedly the skilled counselling and advice Mrs Johns had been able to offer prevented far more serious problems which could have included rifts between Mr and Mrs Floyd, the rejection of Edward and the deep depression of his mother. These achievements rested on Mrs Johns's ability to observe a situation closely, to acknowledge unspoken communications, to accept anger, depression and feelings of failure without being condemning, placatory or full of false reassurance. Her recognition of the differing needs of parents and their children made it possible for her to present Mrs Floyd with various options, and to discourage her from believing that approval and success could come only from conforming to rigidly defined roles. Most important of all, this help was offered in the context of a relationship in which Mrs Floyd could depend on Mrs Johns, value her approval and trust her judgment.

Some problems in counselling

It is widely acknowledged that counselling people who are
unhappy about a pregnancy poses severe strains which make some
unwilling to specialise in this field and others, who cannot
escape contact with pregnant women, avoid serious and prolonged
discussion with them. Counsellors may need to work intensively,
although often for only limited periods, with people in great
distress. Indecision and frequent changes of mind are not uncommon and can be exhausting. Perhaps most important of all,
counsellors have to accept that, although anxieties may be happily
and speedily resolved, there is frequently no simple solution to the
problems which arise when a pregnancy is unwanted. Counsellors
are continually exposed to this suffering. They recognise the deep
regrets of women who wish they had not conceived and who will
bear a child resentfully or with resignation. They are involved with
the agonies of indecision experienced by many families faced with
an unwanted pregnancy. They witness the hardship and unequal
struggles that are a part of the everyday life of those whose
children were unintended and unwanted, and who are given little
support to make a success of their reluctant parenthood. For
counsellors involvement in any way with termination of pregnancy
brings moral doubts or repugnance. Even in those rare instances
where there seems to be a relatively easy and happy way out of
these dilemmas counsellors may not be able to ensure this. Accommodation may be quite unobtainable and welfare benefits
inadequate; abortions are not always readily available; it is not
certain that an adoptive home can be found for a baby, or that a
mother will, when faced with the reality of parting, stand by her
previous decision. The counsellor lives, therefore, in a world of
lesser evils where a huge price may have to be paid for human
ignorance, impetuosity and selfishness. This suffering may last for
years and extend from one generation to another.

Working with people faced with an unwanted pregnancy also
throws into stark relief two of the most central problems in
counselling: that of helping people reconcile what they want with
what is possible, and of the management of counsellors' power
and authority.

Working with ambivalence

The ambivalence with which pregnancy is so often viewed means that answers to the question 'what does this man or woman really want?' can rarely be simple, but must take into account personalities, feelings and social situations. When pregnancy is very much unwanted decisions have to be made which will lead, in the end, to the least pain and the fewest regrets; these cannot be altogether avoided. Acceptance of this complexity, crucial though it is, brings several difficulties. Conflicts may be communicated indirectly; questions which imply that problems may not be as simple as they appear may be greeted with hostile denials; outright acceptance of an individual's strong protestations can bring complaints about counsellors' naivety.

On closer examination these reactions are not surprising. Working with ambivalence means drawing attention to uncomfortable parts of an individual's personality and experience; and in many respects pregnancy is a forcing house of women's ambivalence. Not every woman can accept easily the tender mothering aspects of her personality, although at times she may yearn for these to flourish. Women with a history of rejection, whose histories of emotional relationships are inevitably painful, may face special problems. Acceptance of maternal feelings can also be hard for those women with strong career interests who fear that motherhood will conflict hopelessly with their other commitments. For such women pregnancy can seem a proclamation that they are not quite the people they claimed to be. Painful though it is to examine these conflicts, not to do this may mean ignoring important aspects of individual personality. Problems may therefore be shelved rather than solved.

Power and authority

These complexities in decision-making are compounded by counsellors' power and authority. For ethical and legal reasons parents' own wishes about a pregnancy or a child's future are not the only considerations to be taken into account. The balancing of conflicting interests and the nature of individuals' right to self-determination present medicine, social work and counselling with some of their gravest dilemmas (F. E. McDermott, 1975).

Perhaps the most difficult question counsellors have to tackle is the extent to which parents who provide, or are highly likely to provide, an inadequate upbringing for their children, should have responsibility for them. Ethics, pragmatism and ignorance quickly become confused. Poverty and the lack of appropriate social resources are frequently the principal causes of poor family care; it is unjust to endanger children's futures by failing to intervene in a highly unsatisfactory background. In the all too usual absence of the material resources which might alleviate a family's problems, alternative care for vulnerable children may have to be considered. Given limited knowledge about the development of these children, and the difficulties of assessing the implications of substitute or continued parental care, these decisions must always be extremely complex (Cheetham, 1976). Although most counsellors are not charged with responsibility for making these decisions, all will at some stage have to help men and women reflect on the implications of parenthood. Despite efforts to be objective, and the essential difference between imposing views and pointing out the consequences of behaviour, they are likely to influence the people seeking their help (Halmos, 1969; Foren and Bailey, 1968; Handler, 1968). Some counsellors are quite reconciled to this; others are uneasy because of the high value they attach to people's freedom to make their own decisions, or because they are aware that their own judgment may well be wrong. After all, the history of belief, pseudo-scientific knowledge and fashion in the care of vulnerable children is a long and sad one (Cheetham, 1976).

To reduce the risks of unhelpful or arbitrary influence there is an onus on counsellors to be honest about their own predilections and prejudices, and to examine these in the light of what is known about unwanted pregnancy and its implications (chapter 5). They also need to be clear about their actual, rather than their imagined, responsibilities and about their relationships with those who seek their help.

People in a crisis are more dependent than usual and therefore more susceptible to influence. This presents counsellors with opportunities and with risks. While relationships may be relatively easy to establish, they need to guard against suggesting courses of action to someone who is not in a state to explore their implications, and who feels it is easiest to do what others seem to think is best. Although a very disturbed person may need to have some limits set, it is quite unethical to exploit individuals' temporary dependence in order that they should do what counsellors think is right.

Advice may also be sought from people in authority. Although some counsellors believe they should never give advice, this is too simple a view. Advice is appropriate on those rare occasions when counsellors are in a position to know they are right, and on matters where the outcome is predictable. Advice could therefore be given by doctors about certain kinds of medical treatment; or people might be advised about which agencies they should approach for help with a particular difficulty. However, with more complex problems, to give advice which may not be taken up can complicate relationships. More important when the issues are grave, when people do not know each other well and when human reactions may be infinitely variable, advice may well be ill-informed, and improper, if it leads people to opt out of examining their own difficulties and of responsibility for their actions.

Attitudes towards people in authority, especially doctors, may also complicate counsellors' tasks. Their power may be resented or exaggerated, or it may be assumed that they are remote and hostile and likely to hold uncompromising views. If these feelings seem to be preventing a relationship from developing it may be helpful for counsellors to describe simply and honestly, the nature and extent of their responsibilities and their views and uncertainties on various topics, emphasising, if it is true – and the ethics of counselling demand that it should be – that it is not their business to impose these views on others. Counsellors may also be taken aback to discover that, after a scrupulously fair presentation of the advantages and disadvantages of a particular course of action, people say they have decided to follow their advice, when none had been offered. Such comments as 'since you think it's best, doctor, I'll have an abortion' may be a sign of women's anxiety to avoid the responsibility, and the guilt, of making their own decisions.

There can be no simple or definite guidelines for the management of these infinitely complex relationships of power, authority, dependence, gratitude and hostility but it is helpful to bear in mind the following principles. Despite possible initial relief, people feel ultimately demeaned if responsibility is taken from them; they also have a way of undermining decisions they feel have been imposed upon them. Since the outcome of un-wanted pregnancy must often be a compromise, it must be one that parents feel they can live with. They need therefore, as far as possible, to make their own choices.

Who needs counselling?

If counselling is loosely defined as providing opportunities for individuals to reflect on the nature of their problems and the options before them, then probably all parents unhappy about a pregnancy need this help, and it may often be provided by friends and relatives. However, not everyone finds it easy to admit to anxieties; these may only be revealed in behaviour, and if parents are invited to talk about the pregnancy and their plans after the baby is born. It is therefore worth being alert to the following situations:

1. A referral late in pregnancy for medical or other help, or a referral made by a friend or relative.
2. Emotional flatness and apparent lack of concern about a pregnancy, particularly when this is accompanied by obvious problems.
3. An apparently total lack of interest in the progress of the pregnancy or the baby as an individual before or after birth.
4. A lack of interest in the baby's father.
5. A rejection of contraception.
6. Indications that what parents say about a pregnancy is belied by their actions.

If attempts to explore the possible anxieties of individuals in these circumstances are unsuccessful counsellors may find it helpful to explain why they raised the question. People often feel less guilty if they do not have to take the initiative in discussing their worries. And they are rarely so suggestible as to interpret a question as an indication of what they should be feeling, if they are not feeling this at all.

It is also widely assumed that women requesting an abortion should be offered counselling help. This has been recommended by the Lane Committee, the Select Committee on the Abortion (Amendment) Bill and most recently by the Department of Health and Social Security (1976). The Lane Committee also identified certain groups as likely to be particularly in need of counselling and certain kinds of specialist help. These included young adolescents, especially those still at school; girls from broken homes; those with a history of marked temperamental instability; those who have had a previously induced abortion; the socially handicapped and isolated; mothers who have a handicapped or subnormal child and those who already have as many children as they can support. To this list might be added those who have tried but failed to abort themselves, the bereaved, and parents who have been told that they are likely to have a handicapped child. Sadly, little attention has been paid to fathers' need for counselling, but they should certainly be involved if they are known to be concerned about a pregnancy or about the welfare of their wives or girl-friends.

There is general agreement that counselling should be offered, not imposed, and that it should never become an obligatory process to be endured as a condition of obtaining other kinds of help. As they stand these rules are sensible, but they tend to assume that counselling involves detailed examination, perhaps during several meetings, of all the circumstances which have contributed to an individual's problem, and that it is a discrete activity, separate from other kinds of help. Certainly when this type of counselling is thought appropriate the reasons must be explained, and consent given. However, with the problems that surround unwanted pregnancy, these principles are rarely so clear cut. As soon as a pregnant woman is invited to talk about her anxieties with someone genuinely interested in her feelings and her point of view, and anxious to help, she is being given a kind of counselling. The very complexity of the issues, and the possible solutions to this dilemma, mean that numerous psychological and social factors may have to be taken into account before appropriate plans can be made.

A main contention of this book is that helpful decisions cannot usually be taken without some counselling, by which is meant the opportunity for reflection with an empathetic person who tries to understand the parents' predicament. It does not make sense to ask for consent to this kind of counselling, as distinct from a deliberate process of self-examination which may extend far beyond the problem for which help has been sought. Nor is it possible, with some of the help available when pregnancies are unwanted, to imagine counselling as an optional extra. How could a woman decide whether to offer her baby for adoption, or to keep him or her, in the face of opposition, without some counselling help? In many cases, mere information about services available, although essential, is not enough. Before making a realistic choice people frequently need to discuss their reactions to the options before them. This too can involve counselling, although it may not be recognised as such.

In pondering on this problem of consent to counselling workers need, therefore, to decide how far such a process can be separated from the other help they give; and if they decide that it is largely inseparable, whether they are also able to offer, for those people who wish it, additional help in the exploration of personal problems. These considerations raise fundamental questions about the objectives of the agency and of the individual counsellor. Is it, for example, a basic assumption that a comprehensive service should be offered to help parents make the best possible provisions for themselves and their children, involving, where relevant, relatives and friends? Does the agency have access to resources necessary for such a service? Alternatively, is help intended to be more limited and specific, confined largely to explaining all the alternatives available, and referring to the sources of assistance which seem most appropriate? Does the agency assume that the majority of people consulting it will opt for a certain course of action, for example abortion, or adoption, or help with keeping a child? If so, how do these assumptions influence counsellors' work?

Not only do counsellors themselves need to be clear about their principal objectives of their agencies, they also need to explain these to the people who seek their help. Without such explanations there can be all kinds of misunderstandings, bitterness and sheer waste of time, perhaps especially in those organisations whose objectives are limited, or where there is a strong commitment to a particular standpoint, for example that abortion is never, or is frequently, a reasonable solution to the problems of unwanted pregnancy.

Timing and duration of counselling

It would be foolish to suggest an ideal or average time-span for counselling. As people vary in their needs and in the time they are willing to spend in discussion, so do counsellors vary in their skill and in the time they have available. They often have to do as much as they can, in full recognition that this is inadequate. There are, nevertheless, some generalisations which can usefully be made. The first is that an anxious woman needs counselling as early as possible in pregnancy. Even if the first discussion cannot be long she will be helped by a speedy offer of an appointment. If she is in a particularly disturbed state she will be reassured to know that she can ask for help between her fixed sessions and that some time, however brief, will be available to her. Her demands are unlikely to be long lasting and her problems more quickly resolved if she has this fairly intensive help.

Many people decide independently when to withdraw from counselling, although ideally this should be a decision reached jointly with the counsellor. However, in sorting out priorities counsellors often have to make their own decisions about the amount of time they can give particular individuals. Helpful considerations to bear in mind are their reactions to stress, their grasp of reality and their capacity for problem solving. An assessment based on these factors will probably give a much more accurate indication of needs than any objectively defined category to which a person belongs.

The question of allocation of time must be related to the depth at which a counsellor hopes to work. Fifteen years ago Caplan (1961) anticipated the now commonly held view that, while it is accepted that early experiences greatly influence later behaviour, it is not usually necessary to probe too deeply into these to help people in a crisis. Their present behaviour, including their response to counselling, provides a reasonable indication of their problems and their capacity for dealing with these. It may also be more helpful to focus on strength and ability to cope and survive rather than dwelling on difficulties. The special characteristics of pregnancy make this style of helping particularly relevant (chapter 3). Although there are people who are so trapped by their past and so crippled by their present circumstances that they will need specialist and long-term help, they are the minority.

This approach does not mean that people should not be helped to relate their past and present experiences; this is an essential part of understanding behaviour. It does, however, mean that it is more usually the task of counsellors to prompt than to probe, to use what they see before them as an aid to understanding. It means guarding against collecting information that neither counsellors nor the people they are trying to help can really use. This is easier for more experienced counsellors, and it is inevitable that those who have not worked much with the problems of unwanted pregnancy will need to go more slowly and to ask more questions. It is important that they do this because the familiarity of pregnancy and parenthood makes it easy for counsellors to generalise from their own experiences. Here as so often in counselling, honesty pays dividends. There is no shame in asking parents to help in elucidating their problems. They are far less likely to feel the object of impertinent or irrelevant enquiry if they know why questions are being asked. The people we try to help have much to teach us; they have a right to know this.

Counselling women considering an abortion

The purpose of counselling is to ensure that the decisions by the two medical practitioners and particularly by the woman herself are taken in the light of all relevant facts about her situation and about the alternatives to termination which are available to her (DHSS, *Circular on Counselling*, 1976, p. 1).

In spite of general agreement about the importance of counselling for those considering an abortion the help available is extremely variable. The problems in providing adequate counselling arise partly from ignorance about the aetiology of unwanted pregnancy, partly because abortion is a highly contentious and emotional subject, and partly because of the short time available for making decisions. It is helpful to see how these difficulties affect doctors, since they must be consulted by every woman who requests an abortion.

The doctor's dilemma

Because the criteria set out in the Abortion Act for the legal termination of pregnancy can be widely interpreted doctors have to work out their own personal frame-work for making decisions, to take into account both the needs of the women, as they perceive them, and their own ethical and medical principles (chapter 6). Since it is assumed that not all requests for abortion will be granted most doctors feel they have to decide which women have 'a good case'.

What is 'a good case'? Horobin *et al.* (1973) have shown how, in the absence of firm medical indications and definite predictable consequences, particularly of refusal to terminate a pregnancy, decisions are inevitably fairly arbitrary. How can doctors judge, with any precision, whether the continuation of an unwanted pregnancy will cause a marriage to break down, or a woman to abandon forever her career and ambitions? The most careful doctor cannot reasonably take responsibility for such long-term eventualities. They therefore commonly resort to their own value judgments and theories about the causes of unwanted pregnancy, and may openly acknowledge the moral perspective of their decision-making. Some women, for example, those who have become pregnant in spite of the conscientious use of contraception, may be thought to 'deserve' an abortion more than the thoughtless or the irresponsible. Refusal to terminate a pregnancy may therefore be punitive, to prevent some women thinking 'they can get away with it'. Decisions are frequently not based on an objective analysis of an individual's problem but on other factors leading the doctor to feel sympathetic. And it is easier to sympathise with someone whose circumstances you can readily understand and with whom you can identify. An interesting example of this partiality is Horobin's findings that, amongst those women asking for a second abortion, the requests of half the nurses were granted compared with only 8 per cent of other women.

To these considerable problems may be added the pressures on doctors to ration abortion, although usually on a somewhat uncertain basis. Rationing may be thought necessary because of shortage of resources, either in the shape of beds, or time, or the co-operation of other staff (chapter 5). There may also be less obvious pressures, such as doctors' fears that too many, or too few, abortions will scandalise the public. Doctors may feel that it is their responsibility to promote social change or to safeguard their perception of conventional sexual morality, and in so far as such matters are linked with the termination of unwanted pregnancy, they can certainly have some influence in these areas.

Patients' reactions

> The patient's pressuring attempts at controlling the doctor would lead him either to argue and fight for his rights or to buy peace by agreeing to abortion. Either way he was on unsure ground and was left feeling insulted or used (Main, 1971, p. 55).

A principal concern of those who have responsibility for discretionary decisions is how to respond to pressures for services which are increasingly seen as a right rather than an exceptional response to certain, usually ill-defined needs. With abortion, because the law is uncertain and there is anyway considerable ignorance of it, and because an unwanted pregnancy is not seen as an illness about which lay people have little knowledge and so no worthwhile opinion, doctors frequently meet women who have taken the initiative in diagnosing their problems and selecting the solution. They may be outspoken in their criticism of what they perceive to be doctors' unfair or inconsistent treatment and whether deliberately or not, they may apply various pressures to get the decision they want. Many doctors are incensed by such 'brazen' behaviour and feel that it diminishes their standing as a responsible professional people. It certainly brings into the open a new kind of relationship between patient and doctor, in which patients tend to define their own needs and doctors' expertise and authority is increasingly recognised as being limited to specific areas.

This relationship has certainly not arisen because of the Abortion Act. It is one consequence of better education, greater affluence and a welfare system which gives certain benefits as a right, thus reducing unquestioning dependence on the good will of professionals. It is part of a profound change in society which Fox (1974) has identified as 'the challenge to officially constituted or conventional authority which increasingly displays itself in politics, in religious hierarchies, in universities and schools and in the family and . . . in the organisations of work' (preface).

Nevertheless, an uninhibited request for an abortion seems particularly challenging to some doctors, partly because they see termination of pregnancy as a profoundly serious matter, partly because of the inevitable insecurity involved in decision-making, and possibly also because some male doctors find it threatening and distasteful for women to take such a bold initiative. Other doctors, while relatively at ease with these direct requests, are thoroughly upset by tears, emotional scenes and threats of suicide. And for some, the passive, seemingly apathetic woman is the greatest challenge because her lack of response gives no clue about the most satisfactory treatment. Her apparent willingness to be pushed around by her relations, and by doctors, presents them with enormous dilemmas about the extent of their authority.

Given all these difficulties it is not surprising that some doctors opt out of attempts at rational problem solving and adopt various stances to protect them from conflict (Ingram, 1971). They may thus decide to agree to all requests for abortion, without examining these in any detail, or they may agree to none, except when a pregnancy gravely threatens a woman's life. In this way they avoid the discomfort of argument and the anxiety of complex decision-making. Hospital doctors are likely to escape the pains and pleasures of witnessing the consequences of these stances.

Time and place of consultations

Some of the greatest difficulties in counselling arise in hospitals where, at least at first sight, it can seem administratively sensible to concentrate this help. It is therefore worthwhile examining these aspects of the organisation of counselling services which can critically influence their quality.

The problems already described are compounded if women have had limited or no discussion with counsellors before their first appointment with a hospital doctor. They may therefore know little about the law relating to abortion, hospital clinic procedures, the medical treatment involved and its possible risks. They frequently have to explain a complicated sequence of events and intimate matters in a very short space of time with someone they do not know. Those who want to take a long cool look at their situation will almost certainly be disappointed, and some women feel compelled to describe their plight in ways designed to attract the sympathy of a doctor, or to pressure him into agreeing to what they want. It is therefore not surprising that women asking for abortions are said to be disruptive, liable to cause a scene if their request is refused and to create a tense atmosphere in a normally brisk and cheerful environment.

There are two main ways of easing these pressures and using resources more efficiently. The first is to arrange out-patient clinic appointments in such a way as to ensure that doctors and patients know that they have time for longer consultations than usual. This is sometimes done by organising special clinics for women who are unhappy about their pregnancies or by timing their appointments for the end of clinic sessions. But however appointments are manipulated, and limited resources may anyway make this impossible, a hospital out-patient clinic is not generally the most appropriate place to discuss all the matters relevant to an abortion request. Apart from the obvious pressures on patients and staff, information hurriedly gathered in a strange atmosphere is almost bound to be inaccurate or misleading. It is therefore more helpful if a woman can be counselled and her situation assessed before she comes to the hospital.

This can be done by general practitioners, health visitors, social workers or lay counsellors. Since the majority of women requesting abortions consult their general practitioners between the seventh and tenth week of gestation, counselling will not seriously reduce the chances of performing an abortion before the twelfth week of pregnancy. It could be offered in the usual two or three weeks' wait for a hospital appointment. Indeed, some doctors find it helpful, when faced with an anxious and possibly manipulative woman, to say immediately that they will arrange a hospital consultation. Once this has been established a woman will probably be more able to look at her situation calmly, and to acknowledge any doubts she may have, without fearing that the expression of ambivalence will lead to her doctor's refusal to consider abortion any further (McCance and McCance, 1971). Should hospital referral prove to be inappropriate, it is easier to cancel appointments at short notice than to arrange them.

With this help women will be reasonably well informed and relatively calm at the time of their hospital consultations. The medical and social information needed by hospital doctors can also be readily available. They are therefore relieved of the total burden of calming, informing and examining, and can confine themselves to discussing those matters they think are most important.

Such an arrangement means that hospital doctors must feel they can rely on community-based staff, and frequently on people who are not doctors, to provide adequate information. But they need not fear that relieving themselves of some of the work of assessment will remove their responsibility for making a decision. It will mean only that these decisions will be better informed, and possibly better understood, by the woman concerned. A further advantage is that patients' continued social and medical care is more likely when relationships have been established with community-based workers. Although with this scheme there would be an overall increase in the responsibilities of community-based workers, their much greater number means that, given proper organisation, they can be carried more easily by them than by hospital personnel.

The content of counselling

To construct a long list of matters which may need to be discussed when parents are considering an abortion would mean repeating much about the circumstances surrounding unwanted pregnancy and the principles of counselling. Simms (1973) has also written lucidly on this subject and the brevity of her booklet makes it especially helpful for busy counsellors. The more important issues for discussion will therefore be only briefly outlined. It may well be possible to deal with these in a short period of concentrated counselling.

First, every woman, and ideally her husband or partner, should be helped to discuss the circumstances leading to the pregnancy and its meaning for the couple. Without this discussion it is difficult to decide on the most appropriate help. This exploration does not have to be long and complicated. For instance, the normally efficient contraception used by a woman who had decided definitely that she does not want any more children may have failed; in this case one of her greatest needs may be to discuss the possibility of sterilisation. On the other hand, a request for abortion may be preceded by much more complex situations, such as those of Jill and Mrs Everett.

Second, parents should be helped to look at the alternatives to abortion, not as an argument against this, but as a part of the attempt to ensure that, in being fully informed, they make the decision which will leave them with the fewest regrets. They also need to know about the statutory and voluntary services which could provide a measure of support.

Third, women need information about the law relating to abortion, the procedures for termination of pregnancy, the likelihood or otherwise of complications, and the availability of after-care. When it seems likely that a woman will go to a hospital where the staff dislike being involved with therapeutic abortions it may be helpful for her to be prepared for this.

Fourth, contraception should be discussed. This is particularly important since so many women having abortions have not practised contraception successfully, or at all. When a woman or a couple are already committed to contraception this discussion may only involve explanation of different methods. For the more ambivalent it may mean looking at their feelings about sexuality and their sexual relationships, and at their attitudes to contraception (chapter 6). It is usually helpful if discussion about contraception remains a constant theme in counselling because women may at first be frightened to admit their failure in contraceptive practice, or they may deny that this is a relevant subject since they never intend to have sexual relations again. Such a reaction is particularly common after an abortion and so this may well be the worst time to introduce the subject of contraception.

Counselling school-age girls

Because pregnancy in the very young usually represents a serious crisis and arouses deep emotional responses there are special problems in counselling this age group.

Perhaps the most important of these centre around the fact that pregnancies of very young girls prompt panic reactions. Very often their parents, friends and doctors think immediately and only of abortion, followed by a resolve to break up the relationship which led to the pregnancy. There is in fact no reason why decisions about these girls' pregnancies should be made any more quickly than about the pregnancies of older women; and there is every reason to provide the highest quality of counselling help.

Unhelpful though they may be, it is not difficult to understand these panic reactions. In Western society the prospect of motherhood for a schoolgirl is quite alien and the chances of her being able to give a child adequate care are very remote, despite the support of her family. Even if grandparents provide a home for the baby numerous problems are likely to remain (chapter 4).

Although pregnancy and motherhood, even if only experienced briefly, will usually mean painful emotional problems for a young girl it does not necessarily follow that the best course of action is to take decisions and to behave in ways which appear almost to deny the fact of the pregnancy, and therefore the circumstances which contributed to it. Such denials, although intended to help the girl, are often more a protection for her family. It is not uncommon for people to look on abortion, as they used to look on adoption, as the end of the problem, as an excuse for ignoring a girl's feelings and difficulties, and as a way of avoiding any discussion of these.

These demands may also reflect parents' unwillingness to recognise their daughter's search for greater independence, their grief that she can no longer be only 'a little girl', and possibly also their jealousy of her now obvious sexuality. They may maintain that the pregnancy was a result of the seduction of an innocent girl, an assertion which is often accompanied by calls for vengeance on the man involved. While seduction is not impossible, it is unusual and these claims more often mask parents' guilt at their failure to control their daughter and to provide her with the security that might have prevented her seeking compensation elsewhere.

For the girl these accusations can hinder her search for identity and threaten her relationship with her boyfriend, a relationship which may be valuable for both of them. Even so, girls may themselves unwittingly collude with such denials. Although some staunchly assert their independence, it is not uncommon for young pregnant girls to seem extremely passive, withdrawn and apparently apathetic about the future. While this behaviour may have led them to become involved in relationships where they were exploited, it may also be a reaction to the pregnancy and the fury it has aroused. Seriously frightened, faced with apparently insoluble problems and surrounded by highly emotional adults, apparently intent on protecting everyone from further harm, they may feel that the easiest course is to withdraw and let things happen. For parents and counsellors this apparent apathy may well seem a confirmation that they have a right and duty to make speedy decisions on the girl's behalf.

Even when girls are not so passive their immatuity must lead those who care for them to wonder how far it is right to allow them to make decisions which will affect the whole course of their lives. Adolescents' frequent lack of confidence may lead them to subscribe to ideologies, and to identify with people quite alien to their parents' world. Adults may rightly suspect that these preoccupations will eventually be discarded, but to try and force this process is usually counter-productive. They are left, therefore, with the problems of trying to help a girl, and perhaps her boyfriend as well, reach a decision which will be least in conflict with her circumstances, and with her emerging personality, at a time when all these things will be more than usually in a state of flux. What guidelines may help the counsellor in such a situation?

Work with parents.

It is extremely important for both the girl, her boyfriend and their parents to be given an opportunity for discussion apart from each other. The expression of painful feelings can be cathartic, but discussions between the different parties are unlikely to be helpful when they are dominated by an emotional atmosphere. People need, therefore, to have some time on their own. These private discussions may help the counsellor understand better and therefore, sympathise more with the dilemmas of each individual affected by the pregnancy. When a young girl becomes pregnant it is easy to identify strongly with one or two individuals to the exclusion of others. Faced frequently with an onslaught of rage, recrimination and apparent hypocrisy, it is the young girl, and perhaps her boyfriend, who seems most in need of understanding and protection. This analysis may well be right, but much work will be undermined if parents feel both misunderstood and disliked. However inadequate the care they have given their children, however two-faced their standards of morality, however selfish their concerns, their daughter's pregnancy is still a painful shock which threatens to shatter their image of themselves and their family. There is little chance that parents will reassess their view of the world and their most important relationships while they feel attacked, not only by their children but by those who are said to be helping them.

Not all parents are in open conflict with their pregnant daughters, and given the extent of sexual relationships amongst young people it is unlikely that pregnancy in young girls can now always be associated with gross problems in family life. Such an event can occur in families where relationships are warm and well-established and may have been prompted by some temporary period of stress. Nevertheless, the pregnancy will inevitably give rise to much sadness and heart searching and everyone involved will need help in re-establishing self-confidence.

Just as parents may be worried about their children's private discussions with counsellors, so may young people be reluctant for their counsellors to meet their parents alone, even when the family knows about the pregnancy. Such a contact may challenge the stereotyped image of inadequate home life often presented by teenagers under stress; and there may be anxieties that the counsellor may cease to be sympathetic once their shortcomings are revealed by their parents. Young people may also fear, when they have made a definite decision about a pregnancy, that this, and therefore their own equilibrium, will be threatened by parental intervention.

This firm attempt to individualise all those involved in the crisis of the pregnancy arises from the belief that however passive, childish and dependent young people may seem, and however tempting it is to give quantities of advice and direction, and to collude unquestioningly with their parents' plans, young people should be given every encouragement to think about their own dilemmas and to make their own decisions. This is a step towards maturity, and their families need to recognise this and so accord them some responsibility and some dignity.

The acceptance of pain

In working with young people, perhaps more than with any other group, it has to be remembered that painful experiences can be a part of emotional development. They are only destructive if they are ignored or denied and people are left without understanding, sympathy or support. A young girl swept into an abortion, with little chance of discussion of the circumstances of pregnancy and its meaning for her, may be left with feelings of great inadequacy. Her sexuality has led to disaster and the apparent implication that, for her, motherhood is an impossibility. The abortion is intended to return her to the state she was in before the crisis of the pregnancy, a state which, although perhaps acceptable to her family, may have been the source of considerable unhappiness for her. What image will such a girl have of her relationships with men and her capacity, at some future date, to be a mother? Provided she, her family and her boyfriend are given proper support, young girls will be far better helped if they can express the complicated tangle of rage, grief, and recrimination which so frequently surround an unintended pregnancy, and can talk about their fantasies of themselves as women and mothers.

It can be especially important to demonstrate acceptance of a girl's potential for successful motherhood if she decides on adoption. This may be achieved if those young mothers who want to do this care for their infants, and have the opportunity to talk about the emotions this arouses in them (Gough, 1964 and 1966). Strongly to discourage, or, worse still, to prevent a girl from temporarily looking after her baby may mean denying her the chance of expressing a vital part of her personality, thus stunting her future emotional development. A girl needs a happy memory of these periods of commitment to her infant, however brief these may have been. She needs to know that she was capable of loving and caring and that those close to her accept this fact. On the other hand there are inevitably risks that this temporary care will make future partings more difficult. Such experiences can become a tender trap from which neither the mother nor her helpers can escape if they allow themselves to be overwhelmed by emotion and sentimentality. Failing to distinguish between a girl's needs and capabilities could mean allowing her to take on responsibilities far beyond her. In fact, Gough found that the very deprived young girls he worked with seemed to be quite aware of the temporary, almost play-acting quality of their maternal care, but nevertheless derived satisfaction from the experience. This was a period when girls who had previously been strongly defended became, for a while at least, much in touch with their feelings. The group and individual counselling they received helped them use this to good advantage. All these possibilities have to be borne in mind in helping a girl reach a decision about the care of her infant in the weeks following delivery.

It is hard to witness the mixture of depth of feeling and superficiality which are characteristic of adolescence. And yet for the sake of the mother and her child it is important not to lose touch with either. Counsellors have, therefore, to be scrupulous in asking whether efforts made ostensibly to protect a young girl from pain are, in fact, a form of self-protection.

Confrontation with reality

The shock and emotional turmoil associated with the pregnancies of young girls make it easy to avoid realities. For example, it is not uncommon after an abortion has been arranged for a girl and her parents to refuse to discuss future contraception. In the aftermath of the trauma of the pregnancy both may maintain that there will be no further sexual relations until after marriage. Although this may be said in all sincerity, and is a natural reaction to an unhappy experience, it is certainly possible a girl will eventually resume sexual relationships. While it would be insulting to take no account of her good resolutions, to collude with them completely, by offering no help with contraception, is irresponsible. Sometimes all that can be done is to give basic information about contraception and where help may be obtained. If a girl maintains she wants nothing more to do with boys, this may fall on deaf ears. It is therefore important to try and establish the kind of relationship which helps a girl return to a counsellor should she decide she wants more assistance. This is not always possible, and if counsellors think they are seen as hostile or remote it may be useful to involve an organisation where young people are specially trained to give informal advice and help to their peers about contraception, venereal disease and sexual problems. Preliminary evaluation of these experimental schemes suggest that they may be far more effective in reaching young people than many professionals.

Denials of any future sexual relations outside marriage may also provide the opportunity for discussing the guilt and sadness which seem so far to have shrouded them, and for helping young people to think more clearly about the ethics of their future relationships, the pleasures and the problems they anticipate. Parents too may need help in accepting their children's progress to adulthood, an acceptance which is all the more difficult if it means coming to terms with their own unhappy experiences of sexuality.

An even more difficult reality to accept may be the inadequate love and care parents have given their children, and the thoughtlessness and selfishness which characterise the behaviour of many adolescents. Awareness of these failings lurks beneath every assertion of innocence and casting of blame. When they come to the surface, as they almost always do if the counsellor has not colluded with the general condemnation of others to which frightened people resort, it may be tempting to make little of them, lest pain and guilt be increased. This is unhelpful. Human failings are a reality; to deny this deprives people of the dignity of responsibility for their behaviour and of the chance to make amends.

In spite of its obvious problems and the emotional upheaval it can mean, the crisis of a young girl's pregnancy may help parents and children deal with tensions in their relationships and draw a family closer together. This is partly because adolescence provides an opportunity for re-enacting earlier difficulties, and partly because, despite their anger, shame and grief, most parents yearn to help their children and to surround them with love and affection.

Problems of confidentiality

Working with adolescents raises in an especially acute form the problems of confidentiality which are inescapable for all counsellors. Young people in difficulty greatly need their parents' support but this cannot be forthcoming unless they are aware of their problems. It may also be felt that parents will be unsympathetic or punitive, or that knowledge of their children's problems will be an intolerable burden for them. Young people's assessment of the situation may be right or wrong, but even when counsellors, through personal knowledge of their parents, believe it to be incorrect they have to consider very seriously whether to pass on information given in confidence. Most counsellors may try to persuade young people to talk to their parents, or to allow someone else to do this.

This general principle is crucial to effective counselling, and some regard it as absolute. For others serious problems remain. What, for example, should they do when they hear that a young girl has been involved in an incestuous relationship? Failure to inform the police means that they are a party to a criminal offence. A decision not to discuss this with the girl's parents while avoiding, in the short term at least, enormous pain and turmoil, means that a damaging situation may continue without help being made available. More commonly, counsellors wonder what they should do when they learn that a girl under the age of sixteen has had sexual intercourse, because this may mean that an offence has been committed against her.

A girl under the age of sixteen cannot lawfully consent to sexual intercourse, and a man who has had intercourse with her commits a criminal offence. If the girl is over thirteen it is a defence for the man, provided he is under twenty-four years of age, and has not previously been charged with a similar offence, to prove that he believed, on reasonable grounds, that she was more than sixteen. In England and Wales, but not in Scotland, a boy under fourteen is assumed in law to be incapable of sexual intercourse. The older the man the greater is the risk of his prosecution.

Clearly this law is frequently broken and prosecutions are comparatively rare. The police may not be informed because of the shame and embarrassment this may mean; even if they do receive a complaint they may decide not to prosecute if the girl and the boy are close in age and they think that the girl gave her partner every encouragement. However, some parents may, as an act of revenge, inform the police about their daughter's relationship and many young people fear that to admit to having intercourse will mean an inevitable entanglement with the law. They may, therefore, be extremely reluctant to confide in adults.

Although most professional people are likely to decide that it would be unethical, and probably unhelpful, to pass on to parents or to police information about a young person's sexual relationships, it is impossible to be absolutely definite about this. What, for example, should social workers do when they learn that several girls in their care have had intercourse with a man who seems to be exploiting them? And if it seems that a girl is beyond the control of her parents, and on the verge of promiscuity, with all the attendant risks, should they use this information as a basis for taking a Care Order, whereby parental responsibilities are transferred to a Local Authority?

Further problems arise, particularly for doctors, when a girl under sixteen, who in law should have her parents' consent to medical treatment, asks for help with contraception. Probably most doctors would seek a girl's permission to consult her parents, but if this is refused, they have then to decide whether to proceed with the advice or treatment they think necessary to her well-being without her parents' knowledge and consent. Professional medical organisations and the Department of Health and Social Security have advised that in such a situation priority may be given to a girl's medical needs. Although this advice provides doctors with some measure of professional protection, some still feel uncertain about their personal ethical responsibilities. A code of ethics recently adopted by the British Association of Social Workers, in recognising social workers' considerable legal responsibilities, is more equivocal about matters of confidentiality.

The decisions counsellors reach about respecting confidential information will depend partly on the age of the young people involved, partly on the weight they attach to their assumed or actual responsibilities for their welfare, and partly on the seriousness of the situation. On the one hand a betrayal of confidence may drive young people away from their only source of help. On the other hand, counsellors have to consider the reactions of parents, should they discover that they have been excluded from matters seriously affecting their children's welfare. The special moral responsibilities of work with young people mean that the answers to these questions cannot always be clear cut.

Individual counsellors should therefore be aware of their profession's or agency's code of practice, and if they are unable to accept this, or they work independently, they should discuss these problems with a more experienced person. Whatever conclusions counsellors may reach, it is imperative that they do not mislead young people, so drawing from them confidences they may later bitterly regret. If it is an agency's policy never to pass on information without consent, it would be helpful for this to be clearly stated. If an absolute assurance cannot be given, this also must be made clear, together with the reasons for this policy. In these circumstances, should it become necessary for a confidence to be broken, a counsellor should make every effort to explain why this has been done. This will probably mean exposing themselves to anger and recrimination, but in the course of such discussions it is sometimes possible for young people to accept that counsellors have acted in their interests, and for the bonds between them to be re-established.

Working with depressed people

It is common for women who are considering, or who have had, an abortion to experience some depression, although it is rare for this to be incapacitating (chapter 6). This is probably also true of women who have been refused abortions, although there have only been a few studies of these women. Some researchers believe that the most severe reactions are likely to occur in the first trimester of pregnancy.

Little is known about the depression of women whose pregnancies are unintended and unwanted but who do not consider an abortion. However, it is probably safe to assume that it will occur in this group rather more frequently than it does among those women who have planned their pregnancies.

There is also some doubt about the incidence of post-natal depression. It is common for women to feel overwhelmed, weepy and depressed a few days after delivery. Most people recognise these 'blues' and they are expected to last only a short while. At the other end of the scale is the small minority of women who suffer a puerperal psychosis, of which severe depression may be a large component. These women are usually admitted to hospital. In between is an undefined number of women – estimates range from 10 to 70 per cent – who feel depressed for some months after giving birth, but who manage, more or less successfully, to cope with their families, perhaps with the help of anti-depressants and tranquillisers. The plight of these women is becoming more widely recognised, as is the fact that many may need some form of counselling as well as medication.

In summary, therefore, while only a very small minority of women suffer severe depression needing long-term medical intervention, counsellors can expect some depressive reaction from many women who are, or have been, unhappy about their pregnancies. This depression can be associated primarily with the physiological changes of pregnancy or birth, or it may be largely a reaction to the social and emotional stresses which are a common feature of pregnancy and motherhood. Frequently both factors play a part. What can counsellors do to help these women?

Accepting a woman's depression

First of all they should be alert to the possibility of depression. This can be well concealed by women who, for various reasons, believe it is wrong for them to show how ill or low they are feeling. Common symptoms of depression are unusual tiredness, lethargy and apathy, difficulties with sleeping, loss of appetite, weepiness and acute anxiety. Baker (1967) says that the very rationality and self-awareness of many depressed mothers means that their problems are ignored, because it is assumed that people with these attributes can cope with life. This assumption is strengthened by the fact that at least some of the women most prone to post-natal depression seem to be particularly conscientious and responsible people, used to having others rely on them. While it is true that these women probably will cope, this is often at great cost to them and their families.

Women and their relatives may therefore need to know how common, and yet how little recognised, post-natal depression is. It is also helpful for them to be told that it will pass, although perhaps not as quickly as is often expected. Recognition of largely denied unhappiness, toleration of depression, plus the firm assertion that this will not last forever, can bring considerable relief. This kind of reassurance is very different from superficial attempts to cheer someone up. 'We only make fools of ourselves if we offer good cheer' (Winnicott, 1963, p. 5).

It is quite difficult to avoid 'offering good cheer'. Depressed people are not good company; their feelings of worthlessness and misery can be contagious; their apathy and lethargy irritating.

Looking on the bright side, while it probably makes the depressed people feel even more guilty, because this is just what they cannot do, offers some protection for counsellors. Their own feelings, for example, envy of a woman's baby, or guilt about the inadequacies of help already given, may make it difficult to tolerate a depressed woman and to stand by her. And yet it is this acceptance and support which she most needs if her view of herself as a worthless, incompetent person is to be countered.

There is no point in offering false reassurance to a depressed woman. If she is not coping adequately with her home and children she should not be told she is. It should, however, be explained that her incapacity is fully understandable and, provided this is true, unlikely in the long run to be seriously damaging to those close to her. Although depressed women will not fully believe this, these realities should be held before them.

Practical help

There are many aspects of pregnancy and early motherhood which are incapacitating. Tiredness, the emotional and physical shock of a sudden change in role, and sheer inexperience in caring for a child all play their part in compounding a depressed woman's poor self-image. She may, therefore, need various kinds of practical help although she will often find it difficult to accept this lest it should seem a proof of her incompetence. Particularly important is the help which goes some way to reducing her feelings of failure as a mother. If she already has children whom she thinks are being neglected she and they may well be comforted by help which gives them some of the care they are temporarily missing, for example, opportunities for play and outings. An exhausted woman, relieved of some household tasks so that she may sleep for short periods during the day, will be in a better state, despite her depression, to care for her infant. This help is usually recognised as essential for the first two or three weeks after delivery. For a family whose mother is depressed, and whose difficulties in sleeping lead to cumulative exhaustion, this help needs to be continued much longer.

Women whose anxiety leads them to panic about the basic care they are giving their babies may be helped if a counsellor whom they like and accept shares, on a few occasions, some of these tasks with her. It is important to emphasise sharing, because the purpose of this help is not to take over the care of the infant, thus leaving the mother feeling more of a failure, but to make practical suggestions if these seem necessary, to calm and reassure the mother about what she is managing successfully, and to acknowledge openly the sheer difficulty, dreariness and hard work of some aspects of infant care. This is especially important for women who feel inferior because of their inexpertise in tasks traditionally thought to be within her competence, simply because they are women.

It is sometimes suggested that a very depressed woman should have a break from her infant. On the whole, although she may be wise to limit, as far as possible, her other domestic responsibilities, it is now generally believed that it is unhelpful for her to be parted from her baby, even if this means they must both be admitted to hospital. Separation, although it may provide a temporary relief, will also confirm her feelings of failure and guilt, and make the eventual reunion more difficult. It is therefore as well not to suggest a complete separation, even when there are relatives willing to care for the baby, without discussing all the possible advantages and disadvantages with a colleague, and attempting to make a full assessment of the extent of a woman's incapacity. It is usually more helpful for those willing to help to assume only partial responsibility for the infant, and to assist them in the complex task of sharing care with a depressed woman.

Aggression and guilt

Some psychiatrists believe that depression occurs when people who find it hard to express their aggression openly, turn this in on themselves. There is much in early motherhood to exacerbate such a reaction. How can women legitimately feel angry with the many helpful people who flock around them during pregnancy and after delivery? Although they may justifiably be angered by well meaning but inconsistent or unhelpful advice, or by attempts to influence them to behave in ways they find unsympathetic, depressed women lose confidence in their judgment and are apt to feel that they can only be grateful for the help offered and all their other advantages.

It is even more difficult for a woman to admit resentment of her baby. How can she be angry with a helpless infant? How does she deal with the fact that at times she wished the infant did not exist, and that she may have tried to bring this about? And yet the truth is that the blameless baby is one cause of the mother's depression. Counsellors need therefore to help women to express their resentment and anger. They may be considerably relieved if these emotions can be expressed within the context of the relationship where they will not be criticised, or argued with, and where they can come to accept their reactions as, in many respects, natural.

Since depressed women are often struggling with earlier unresolved problems, counsellors may wonder whether this is a good opportunity for examining these at some depth. It is not usually helpful to do this with a woman who is very depressed. This is partly because she will have little energy to spare for such an exercise, and partly because her depression will lead her to interpret her experiences in a gloomy, self-denigrating way, thus exacerbating her depression. At such times it is more productive to see people frequently, but for limited periods. However, women coming out of a depression may begin to think about its various components, and at this stage it can be helpful to discuss those past events and aspects of their personality which may have contributed to their illness (Deykin, 1971). Others will prefer to put the whole episode behind them, and there is no evidence that their recovery is less complete or long lasting than that of the more reflective women.

One of the greatest difficulties of working with depressed people is their profound, although usually unacknowledged, need for strong and caring relationships at a time when they feel least acceptable and least able to contribute to these. At one level depressed people want, and therefore often invite, rejection; this will confirm their badness; they will no longer have to bother. And yet such a rejection can be disastrous. Frequently it is only the faith and commitment of relatives, friends and counsellors that keep a person in touch, at least minimally, with the reality that they are both good and bad, strong and weak, able to love and hate.

Depressed people often believe that their demands are so great that they will drive away those who are trying to help them. It can therefore be helpful for counsellors to explain simply that they know this is what a person feels, that they have been involved with many other depressed people and that they are well able to bear this. A depressed and anxious woman can, for the time, be very dependent, and if this is accepted by a counsellor, it can speed her recovery. Dependence is a sign of her ability to assess the reality of her present incapacity and to entrust herself to another person. It should not be discouraged for fear it will become normal behaviour. It is far more worrying when a woman thinks she is beyond help and so withdraws from human contact.

Such a commitment is frequently more difficult for a woman's relatives. They are more continuously in touch with her, and although they may accept that post-natal depression is an illness, especially if some medical treatment is being given, this does not protect them from anxiety and despair, or from the hostility which a depressed person's apathy and hopelessness arouses. They therefore need as much support as the depressed person and, in particular, help with feelings of guilt they may have if they see themselves as partially responsible for the depression. A husband may bitterly regret contraceptive carelessness, or a mother the burden that her expectations have meant for her daughter.

Witnessing depression and its effects can be a frightening experience and counsellors frequently wonder whether they should call on more specialist help. The following guidelines may be worth considering.

Referral for specialist help

If a depressed woman is not receiving any medical help she should be encouraged to consult her doctor. If she cannot make this effort it may well be appropriate for a counsellor, with permission, to contact her general practitioner and explain the situation, or to encourage her relatives to do this. However, many women remain extremely depressed despite medication and some feel that the apparent failure of their present treatment makes it pointless to seek further medical help. They may also fear the form this might take, for example, admission to hospital or electro-convulsive therapy. When should counsellors try to persuade a woman to return to her doctor, or themselves call in additional help?

It is appropriate to consider such steps if a depression appears to continue unabated, with no positive response to medication, reassurance or support, especially if the burden on relatives seems to be becoming intolerable. It is also important to take seriously a woman's self-destructive or suicidal thoughts. These may be blatant; more usually they take the form of hints and allusions that it can be more comfortable to ignore. But this does not help the woman who may feel that, since her depression is not recognised, she must draw attention to it more directly.

Contrary to· popular belief people do not attempt suicide because someone has put the idea into their heads; most depressed people are only too aware of this possibility. Suicidal behaviour is a sign that they believe there are no other alternatives. Counsellors need, therefore, to make some assessment of the seriousness of suicidal intention, and to decide whether emergency intervention is necessary, or whether a woman's main need is to share the depth of the desperation revealed in her morbid brooding. Those who are not medically qualified should discuss their assessment with a doctor or with a person with considerable experience of work with the psychiatrically ill.

A woman's fears that she may harm her child must also be taken seriously. In the past these fears often met only with reassurance, with little attempt to assess the likelihood of actual harm for the child. A distinction can, of course, be made between a woman's doubts about her ability to care for her offspring adequately and her expressed or implied fears that she will lose control and cause physical harm. Both kinds of anxiety need to be discussed with the woman, and usually also with her husband, but where there is a question of possible harm to the child a counsellor should seriously consider referral to a social services department. Parents likely to need special help, and whose children are particularly vulnerable, are those who were chronically deprived in their own childhood, who are socially isolated and who suffer various kinds of physical strain.

Such a referral raises in an acute form the ethics of confidentiality. Although it is a serious matter for parents' possible inadequacies to become the object of official concern, it is irresponsible to dismiss their insinuations and warnings, thus failing to protect them and their children from the behaviour they fear.

Working with husbands and boyfriends

While lip service is paid to the importance of contacts with the husbands and boyfriends of women unhappy about their pregnancies these occur relatively rarely. There are various reasons for this, including women's unwillingness for their problems to be discussed with anyone else and assumptions that pregnancy is an exclusively female concern, that women should be protected from men, that men will not wish to be involved and that these contacts will serve no useful purpose.

With rare exceptions, counsellors should not approach relatives or friends without the permission of the people who have sought their help. However, some women's reluctance to agree to these contacts is based on a misunderstanding of their purpose. This must, therefore, be carefully explained and the possible advantages and disadvantages honestly examined. Some women may not realise that many counsellors see their job as including some responsibility for working with friends and relatives. They may also assume that no-one else will want to be concerned with their present crisis. Occasionally this assumption is correct; more often it is a product of guilt and embarrassment and anxiety not to be a burden on those who would be willing to help if they knew of the woman's predicament. A girl may also be anxious to protect her boyfriend from criticism or recrimination or, if he is already trying to escape from the situation, to avoid the chance of further rebuff should he refuse to meet the counsellor.

On those rarer occasions when counsellors are urged to meet a boyfriend as part of a woman's plans for revenge and punishment they must explain that although they will certainly contact this person they will not play the role that seems to be envisaged. These meetings often prove fruitful, for when the relative finds his expectations of being treated as a villain are not fulfilled, and he too is offered some understanding and help, he may well be able to respond better to his girlfriend's needs.

A desire to escape financial responsibility for a child is by no means always the main reason for men's reluctance to meet counsellors. Many seem to be more deterred by the fear that they will be criticised and castigated for 'having got a girl into trouble' and be allowed little or no opportunity to present their side of the story, which may include the realistic assessment that, to some extent, 'she asked for it'. They may also be reluctant to approach an organisation which seems formal and remote, whose staff they assume will inevitably side with the girl. This impression may be confirmed when no independent efforts are made to contact a man and he only receives messages relayed by his girlfriend, possibly elaborated to suit her purposes, that 'they' want to see him. When independent contacts with boyfriends have been attempted counsellors have found not only an encouraging response, but also that these men have often felt totally isolated and excluded. They, too, often have problems they need to discuss and may welcome the opportunity to show concern for their girlfriend and for the child. This is not surprising in view of the fact that the majority of single women's pregnancies result from well-established relationships (Yelloly, 1965; Weir, 1968; Williams and Hindell, 1972). It is unhelpful to regard a boyfriend as some kind of hit and run driver. If a man is encouraged to be a refugee from the consequences of his own sexuality, this must surely cast a shadow on his estimation of himself and his future relationships with women. Rowe (1966) and Pochin (1969) have given considerable thought to the opportunities and problems of work with unmarried fathers, and if their suggestions were put into practice the counselling available to these men would certainly improve.

To a lesser extent the difficulties of unmarried fathers apply also to the husbands of women with unwanted pregnancies. If they have done little to prevent a pregnancy, perhaps because they see contraception as the exclusive concern of their wives, they may be guilty or regretful about their own lack of responsibility and frightened that they will be blamed and criticised. The pregnancy may well have caused unhappy arguments and differences of opinion not fully resolved. It is uncomfortable to raise such matters again, although to ignore them may mean fostering resentment damaging to the couple's relationship, and to any child they may have.

If counsellors are to be committed to working with relatives, they need to be clear about their objectives. These will vary according to a counsellor's responsibility and professional concern but the following are worth consideration.

First, if a confused woman needs help in reaching a decision about her pregnancy it is helpful for the counsellor to have as full a picture as possible about her circumstances. Taking account of the woman's actual, or reasonably foreseeable, environment (Abortion Act 1967) usually includes some understanding of her relationship with her close relatives. The quality of these relationships will considerably influence a woman's intention to seek an abortion, to keep her child, or to place him or her for adoption (Yelloly, 1965; Pearson, 1973). Although a woman may think she has presented as fair and as full a picture as possible, the crisis of pregnancy may well contribute to distorted impressions and panic reactions which bear little relation to reality. Without the opportunity for calmer, more reflective discussion the people closest to the woman may well not be regarded as potential sources of help.

Second, contact with relatives means that when a pregnancy is associated with problems in a relationship there is an opportunity for these to be tackled jointly, and for something positive to be derived from a crisis which seemed, at first sight, to mean nothing but disaster.

Finally, although the welfare of the mother and the child should be counsellors' prime concern, it is not their only one. The woman's husband or boyfriend, and, if she is very young, her parents, also have needs and a right to help. Their welfare and that of the woman and her child may well be inseparable. For example, if a man is led to believe that all that is required of him is a financial contribution towards the support of his child, and that he has none of the other responsibilities and rewards of fatherhood, the help he gives may well be only grudging. Alternatively, he may decide relentlessly to assert his rights to custody and access, as a weapon in a long drawn-out battle with the girl and her family with little regard for the welfare of the child. Although it is generally agreed that it is to everyone's advantage if fathers take more than just financial responsibility for their children, the fathers of natural children are rarely encouraged to live up to these expectations. Counsellors might well consider whether, in their own work, they contribute to this confusion.

Some fundamental questions

A remedy cannot be found in undoing social development, but in attempting to find new adjustments to changed conditions, to organise social life in a way which satisfies human needs, emotional no less than economic (Klein, 1946, p. 36).

Viewed within the context of man's whole life on this planet we are witnessing the gathering speed of an ever widening human impulse towards an enhancement of individual life and experience (Fox, 1974, preface).

This chapter, like much of the book, has focused on the immediate problems posed by an unwanted pregnancy, and on ways of resolving these. But there are wider issues on which counsellors need to ponder. Although most individuals feel powerless to bring about profound changes on their own, it does not follow that we are at the mercy of uncontrollable forces in society. Our laws, our customs and our attitudes reflect choices we have made, often in the realisation that they are not ideal, but in the hope that they are better than what has gone before. And as this generation, perhaps more than any other, must realise, the social arrangements which emerge from these choices change rapidly. Changes begin with ideas, and the ideas of those with tried and thoughtful experience of society's problems are especially valuable because they will not be based on simple explanations and simple solutions. To meet their responsibilities as particularly well-informed citizens, counsellors have to bring to public notice the central dilemmas in society, of which unwanted pregnancy is only a symptom.

The first of these dilemmas is the growing realisation that the achievements of a society, not primarily concerned with a struggle for its mere survival, bring in their wake changes scarcely dreamt of by those who strive to improve the conditions of life of their fellow human beings. These achievements have encouraged the boundless aspirations of men and women who believe that happiness on earth, at this present moment, is their right. These beliefs are by no means the prerogative of those who see human destiny as confined to this planet. They are shared by most Christians and others who look to some kind of life after death. How may these aspirations be met? Exploring this same question in another context, that of the management of industrial enterprise, Fox (1974, preface) has written:

Over substantial and ever widening portions of the globe . . . increasing numbers of people are demanding that their allotted span of life should yield them more than a mere slavish and anonymous preoccupation with survival. More and more they become conscious of a self and an identity that seeks nourishment not only through a share in the world's growing economic wealth but also through rising standards of health, education, status, respect, or whatever else they may see as giving meaning to their life.

Human happiness is defined according to the prevailing values in society. Today these extol, and few would wish otherwise, decent and rising material standards of living, the importance of rewarding work and enriching leisure, and the right of individuals to make decisions about the shape of their lives. These values are not diminished by the belief that man's ultimate destiny does not rest in this world. Whether such conditions of life are actually attainable, or whether they bring with them human happiness, matters little beside the crucial fact that they are *seen* as important, even essential goals. This is the context of women's struggles for emancipation, as it is of workers' determination to have a greater share of a nation's wealth.

This pursuit evolves its own rules, many of which challenge fundamentally the unquestioned values of previous generations. One such challenge is the pragmatism which poses these questions: 'what are our responsibilities towards those whose lives seem destined to be unhappy, despite all the efforts of human ingenuity? Is birth or abortion to be preferred? Should parents be encouraged to part with those children for whom they cannot provide adequate care?' No longer are the answers to these questions held to be the province of established authorities, with the right to shape the rules of behaviour of the mass of the population. Men and women now believe their own opinions deserve respect.

These challenges, and the growing pressure for individuals to exert greater control over their own lives and to have freedom in their moral choices, are the inevitable accompaniment to rising educational standards. In an examination of the changing concepts of sexual morality Gill (1971, p. 37) has this to say:

> You cannot educate populations to high levels of knowledge, and to apply first principles to problems in the educational and economic sectors, without their applying the same logico-deductive procedures to their own lives, and hence making their own decisions about what they perceive to be their interests. Under such conditions individuals are increasingly likely to select patterns of sexual behaviour and family size in accordance with their own definitions of what is acceptable.

Gill concludes that in a hedonistic society sexual relations will be idiosyncratic and individualistic. Primarily the concern of the participants, their morality will be defined in terms of the consequences. Contrary to expectation, if these values were widely accepted, unwanted pregnancies might become less common. Explicit recognition of the sexual relationships of the unmarried could encourage the use of contraception. It is the belief that these relationships are morally undesirable that makes contraceptive preparation unlikely (chapters 4 and 6). Nevertheless, it has to be recognised that in sexual relationships, more than in any other sphere, it is impossible to devise ways of eliminating human carelessness, laziness and irresponsibility.

If submission to authority can bring apathy, resentment and unwarranted intrusions into individual liberties, greater freedom of choice brings painful uncertainty and personal responsibility for mistaken decisions. How will women shape their lives? How can counsellors make judgments about an individual's health and happiness? And in an era which extols human rationality, and therefore individual choice, how can we control the selfishness and irrationality which promises the good life for all, but withholds it from many; which, for example, enjoins parents to provide the highest standards for their children, but denies them the means to do this? It would be possible in our society, if we had the will, to ensure a decent standard of living for families with one parent. Women could have a much greater opportunity to pursue the interests and rewards which are now largely the province of men. Poor parents could be given more help to provide adequately for their children. We could also provide the mentally and physically handicapped with an immeasurably better life than is usually their lot. But these are not our priorities, and while they are not we have to live with the logical inconsistencies, the moral ambiguities, and the human unhappiness and conflict which surround unwanted pregnancy and the methods we have evolved for dealing with it.

Your conclusions about these priorities, about the nature of happiness, and about individual freedom and responsibility are needed if conditions are to change. What have you decided?

Bibliography

Abercrombie, M. L. J. (1960), *The Anatomy of Judgement*, Hutchinson, London.

Andry, R. G. (1971), *Delinquency and Parental Pathology*, Staples Press, London.

Arreggar, C. E. (ed.) (1966), *Graduate Women at Work*, Oriel Press, London.

Ashdown-Sharp, P. (1975), *The Single Woman's Guide to Pregnancy and Parenthood*, Penguin, Harmondsworth.

Association of British Adoption Agencies, *Analysis of Adoption and In Service Training Guide*.

Baker, A. (1967), *Psychiatric Disorders in Obstetrics*, Blackwells, Oxford.

Barber, D. (1975), *Unmarried Fathers*, Hutchinson, London.

Bardwick, J. (1973), 'Psychological Factors in the Acceptance and Use of Oral Contraceptives' in J. T. Fawcett (ed.), *Psychological Perspectives on Population*, Basic Books, New York.

Bernstein, R. (1966), 'Are we Still Stereotyping the Unmarried Mother?' in R. Roberts (ed.), *The Unwed Mother*, Harper & Row, London.

Bessell, R. (1971), *Interviewing and Counselling*, Batsford, London.

Bird, B. (1973), *Talking with Patients*, Blackwells, Oxford.

Bone, M. (1973), *Family Planning Services in England and Wales*, HMSO, London.

Bott, E. (1957), *Family and Social Network*, Tavistock, London.

Bowlby, J. (1951), *Maternal Care and Mental Health*, World Health Organisation Monograph no. 2, Geneva.

Bowlby, J. (1969), *Attachment and Loss*, vol. I, *Attachment*, 1969; vol. II, *Separation*, 1973, Hogarth Press, London.

Breen, D. (1975), *The Birth of a First Child*, Tavistock, London.

Briggs Report (1972), *The Report of the Committee on Nursing*, HMSO, London.

British Association of Social Workers (1975), *Analysis of the Children's Bill 1975*.

Callahan, D. (1970), *Abortion: Law, Choice and Morality*, Collier-Macmillan, London.

Caplan, G. (1957), 'Psychiatric Aspects of Maternal Care', *American Journal of Public Health*, vol. 47.

Caplan, G. (1961), *An Approach to Community Mental Health*, Tavistock, London.

Caplan, G. (1970), *The Theory and Practice of Mental Health Consultation*, Tavistock, London.

Cartwright, A. (1970), *Parents and Family Planning Services*, Routledge & Kegan Paul, London.

Cartwright, A. (1976), *How Many Children?* Routledge & Kegan Paul, London.

Cartwright, A. and Lucas, S. (1974), *Survey of Abortion Patients*, Lane Report, vol. 3, HMSO, London.

Cartwright, A. and Waite, M. (1972), 'General Practitioners and Abortion', *Journal of the Royal College of General Practitioners*, Supplement no. 1, vol. 22.

Cheetham, J. (1976), 'Pregnancy in the Unmarried: The Continuing Dilemmas for Social Policy and Social Work' in A. H. Halsey (ed.), *Traditions of Social Policy*, Blackwells, Oxford.

Child Poverty Action Group (1975), *National Welfare Benefits Handbook*, ed. R. Lister.

Church Assembly Board for Social Responsibility (1973), *Abortion: an Ethical Discussion*, Church Information Office, London.

Collins, M. (ed.) (1964), *Women Graduates and the Teaching Profession*, Manchester University Press, Manchester.

Community Relations Commission (1975), *Who Minds? A Study of Working Mothers and Child minding in Ethic Minority Communities*.

Coote, A. and Gill, T. (1974), *Women's Rights: A Practical Guide*, Penguin, Harmondsworth.

Crellin, E. *et al.* (1971), *Born Illegitimate: Social and Educational Implications*, National Foundation for Educational Research in England and Wales.

Cutter, M. (ed.) (1974), *Housing Rights Handbook*, Shelter.

Dahlstrom, E. (1967), *The Changing Roles of Men and Women*, Duckworth, London.

De Beauvoir, Simone (1953), *The Second Sex*, Jonathan Cape, London.

Department of Employment and Productivity Manpower Paper no. 11 (1974), *Women and Work*, HMSO, London.

Department of Employment and Productivity Manpower Paper no. 11 (1975), *Women and Work*, HMSO, London.

Department of Health and Social Security (1974), *The Family in Society: Preparation for Parenthood*, HMSO, London.

Deutsch, H. (1946), *The Psychology of Women*, 2 vols, Research Books, London.

Deykin, G. Y. (1971) 'Treatment of Depressed Women', *British Journal of Social Work*, vol. 1, no. 3.

Dinnage, R. and Pringle, M. K. (1967), *Residential Care: Facts and Fallacies*, Longmans, London.

Drabble, M. (1972), *The Millstone*, Penguin, Harmondsworth.

Draper, E. (1972), *Birth Control in the Modern World*, Pelican, Harmondsworth.

Eppel, E. M. and Eppel, M. (1966), *Adolescents and Morality*, Routledge & Kegan Paul, London.

Figes, E. (1970), *Patriarchal Attitudes*, Faber & Faber, London.

Finer Report (1974), *Report of the Committee on One-Parent Families*, 2 vols, HMSO, London.

Fogarty, M. P., Rapoport, R. and Rapoport, R. N. (1971), *Sex, Career and Family*, Allen & Unwin, London.

Foren, R. and Bailey, R. (1968), *Authority in Social Casework*, Pergamon, London.

Forssman, H. and Thuwe, I. (1966), 'One Hundred and Twenty Children born after Application for Therapeutic Abortion Refused', *Acta Psychiatric Scandinavia*, vol. 42.

Fox, A. (1974), *Man Mismanagement*, Hutchinson, London.

Fraser, R. (1968), *Work*, vol. 1, Penguin, Harmondsworth.

Friedan, B. (1971), *The Feminine Mystique*, Victor Gollancz, London.

Gavron, H. (1968), *The Captive Wife*, Penguin.

George, M. D. (1925), *London Life in the Eighteenth Century*, Kegan Paul, Trench & Trubner, London.

George, V. (1970), *Foster Care: Theory and Practice*, Routledge & Kegan Paul, London.

Gill, D. G. (1971), 'Changing Patterns of Sexual Behaviour and Adjustment', unpublished paper.

Gough, D. (1964), *Schoolgirl Unmarried Mothers*, NCUMC, London.

Gough, D. (1966), *Pregnancy in Adolescence: the Very Young Mother*, NCUMC, London.

Greenwood, W. (1975), *Love on the Dole*, Penguin, Harmondsworth.

Greer, G. (1971), *The Female Eunuch*, Paladin, London.

Halmos, P. (1969, *The Faith of the Counsellors*, Constable, London.

Halsey, A. H. (ed.) (1972a), *Trends in British Society*, Macmillan, London.

Halsey, A. H. (1972b), *Educational Priority*, HMSO, London.

Handler, J. (1968), 'The Coercive Children's Officer', *New Society*, 3 October 1968.

Hart, H. L. A. (1972), 'Abortion Law Reform: The English Experience', *Melbourne University Law Review*, vol. 8, no. 3, 1972.

Heinicke, C. M. and Westheimer, I. J. (1966), *Brief Separations*, Longmans, London.

Hindell, K. and Grahame, H. (ed.) (1974), *Out Patient Abortion*, Pregnancy Advisory Service, London.

Holman, R. (1970), *Unsupported Mothers*, Mothers in Action, London.

Holman, R. (1973), *Trading in Children*, Routledge & Kegan Paul, London.

Holman, R. (1975), 'Unmarried Mothers, Social Deprivation and Child Separation', *Policy and Politics*, vol. 3, no. 4, June.

Horobin, G. W., et al. (1973), *Experience with Abortion: A Case Study in North-East Scotland*, Cambridge University Press.

Houghton Report (1972), *Report of the Departmental Committee on the Adoption of Children*, HMSO, London.

Hunt, A. (1968), *A Survey of Women's Employment*, vols I and II, HMSO, London.

Hunt, A., Fox, J. and Morgan, M. (1973), *Families and their Needs*, HMSO, London.

Hutt, C. (1972), *Males and Females*, Penguin, Harmondsworth.

Illsley, R. and Gill, D. G. (1968), 'Changing Trends in Illegitimacy', *Social Science and Medicine*, vol. 2, Pergamon.

Illsley, R. and Hall, M. H. (1975), *Psycho-Social Aspects of Abortion: A Review of Issues and Needed Research*, WHO Bulletin, Nov.

Illsley, R. and Hall, M. H. (1974), 'Post Abortion Counselling', unpublished paper.

Ingham, C. and Simms, M. (1972), 'Study of Applicants for Abortion at the Royal Northern Hospital, London', *Journal of Biosocial Science*, vol. 4.

Ingram, I. M. (1971), 'Abortion Games – an Inquiry into the Working of the Act'. *The Lancet*, 30 Oct.

Jackson, B. (ed.) (1976), *Action Register Three*, National Educational Research and Development Trust, London.

Jaffee, B. and Fanshel, D. (1970), *How They Fared in Adoption – A Follow Up Study*, Columbia University Press, New York.

Jephcott, P., Seear, N. and Smith, J. (1962), *Married Women Working*, Allen & Unwin, London.

Kadushin, A. (1970), *Adopting Older Children*, Columbia University Press, New York.

Kaig, L. and Nilsson, A. (1972), 'Emotional and Psychotic Illness Following Childbirth' in J. E. Howells (ed.), *Modern Perspectives in Psycho-Obstetrics*, Oliver & Boyd, Edinburgh.

Kellmer-Pringle, M. L. (1966), *Adoption Facts and Fallacies*, Longmans, London.

Kitzinger, S. (1962), *The Experience of Childbirth*, Victor Gollancz, London.

Klein, J. (1965), *Samples from English Cultures*, vols I and II, Routledge & Kegan Paul, London.

Klein, V. (1946), *The Feminine Character, History of an Ideology*, Routledge & Kegan Paul, London.

Klein, V. (1965), *Britain's Married Women Workers*, Routledge & Kegan Paul, London.

Kleinmann, R.L. (1971), *Family Planning for Midwives and Nurses*, International Planned Parenthood Federation, London.

Lafitte, F. (1972), *Abortion in Britain Today*, British Pregnancy Advisory Service, London.

Lafitte, F. (1975), *The Abortion Hurdle Race*, British Pregnancy Advisory Service, London.

Lambert, J. (1971), 'Survey of 3,000 Unwanted Pregnancies', *British Medical Journal* 156, 16 Oct.

Lambert, L. and Rowe, J. (1973), *Children Who Wait*, Association of British Adoption Agencies, London.

Lane Report (1974), *Committee of Inquiry into the Working of the Abortion Act*, vols 1, 2 and 3, HMSO, London.

Lewis, S. C. *et al.* (1971), 'Out Patient Termination of Pregnancy', *British Medical Journal*, 4 Dec.

Lomas, P. (1967), 'The Significance of Post-Partum Breakdown' in *The Predicament of the Family*, P. Lomas (ed.), Hogarth, London.

Luker, K. (1976), *Taking Chances: Abortion and the Decision not to Contracept*, University of California Press, Berkeley and London.

Lynes, T. (1974), *Guide to Supplementary Benefits*, Penguin, Harmondsworth.

McCance, C. and Hall, D. J. (1972), 'Sexual Behaviour & Contraceptive Practice of Unmarried Female Undergraduates at Aberdeen University', *British Medical Journal*, 17 June.

McCance, C. and McCance, P. F. (1971), 'Abortion or No Abortion – What Decides?', *Journal of Biosocial Science*, vol 3.

McDermott, F. E. (1975), *Self Determination in Social Work*, Routledge, Kegan Paul, London.

Macintyre, S. (1976a), 'To Have or to Have Not – Promotion and Prevention of Childbirth in Gynaecological Work' in M. Stacey (ed.), *Sociological Review Monograph*.

Macintyre, S. (1976b), 'Who Wants Babies? The Social Construction of Instincts' in S. Allen and D. Barker (ed.), *Dependence and Exploitation: Process and Change*, Tavistock, London.

McWhinnie, A. M. (1967), *Adopted Children: How They Grow Up*, Routledge & Kegan Paul, London.

Maddox, B. (1975), *The Half Parent*, André Deutsch, London.

Main, T. F., (1971), 'Asking for Abortion', *Family Planning*, vol. 20, no. 3, Oct.

Mandell, B. (1973), *Where are the Children?*, Lexington Books, Mass.

Marsden, D. (1969), *Mothers Alone*, Allen Lane, The Penguin Press, London.

Mead, M. (1954a), *Male and Female*, Gollancz, London.

Mead, M. (1954b), 'Some Theoretical Considerations on the Problem of Mother Child Separation', *American Journal of Orthopsychiatry*, vol. XXIV, no. 3, July.

Medawar, M. and Pyke, D. (ed.) (1971), *Family Planning*, Penguin, Harmondsworth.

Menzies, I. E. P. (1960), 'A Case Study in the Functioning of Social Systems as a Defence against Anxiety', *Human Relations*, vol. 13, no. 2.

Mill, J. S. (1957), *On Liberty*, Everyman edn, Dent, London.

Millard, D. W. (1971), 'The Abortion Decision', *British Journal of Social Work*, vol. 1, no. 2, Summer.

Millett, K. (1971), *Sexual Politics*, Rupert Hart Davis, London.

Mitchell, J. (1971), *Woman's Estate*, Penguin, Harmondsworth.

Mitchell, J. (1974), *Psycho-analysis and Feminism*, Allen Lane, The Penguin Press, London.

Myrdal, A. and Klein, V. (1968), *Women's Two Roles*, Routledge & Kegan Paul, London.

National Council for the Unmarried Mother and Her Child (NCUMC) (now National Council for One Parent Families), *Annual Report*, 1972-73.

Newson, J. and Newson, E. (1965), *Patterns of Infant Care in an Urban Community*, Penguin, Harmondsworth.

Newson, J. and Newson, E. (1970), *Four Years Old in an Urban Community*, Penguin, Harmondsworth.

Nicholson, J. (1968), *Mother and Baby Homes*, Allen & Unwin, London.

Noonan, J. T. (1970), *The Morality of Abortion*, Harvard University Press, America.

Norman, J. F. (1969), *Banana Boy*, Secker & Warburg, London.

North, M. (1972), *The Secular Priests*, Allen & Unwin, London.

Nye, Wan F. and Hoffman, L. W. (1963), *The Employed Mother in America*, Rand McNally, Chicago.

Oakley, A. (1972), *Sex, Gender and Society*, Temple Smith, London.

Oakley, A. (1974a), *Housewife*, Allen Lane, The Penguin Press, London.

Oakley, A. (1974b), *The Sociology of Housework*, Martin Robertson, London.

Parker, R. (1966), *Decision in Child Care*, Allen & Unwin, London.

Parker, T. (1972), *In No Man's Land*, Panther, London.

Parsons, T. and Bales, R. F. (1964), *Family, Socialisation and Interaction Process*, Free Press, New York.

Pearson, J. F. (1973), 'Social and Psychological Aspects of Extra Marital First Conceptions', *Journal of Biosocial Science*, Oct.

Peck, E. (1973), *The Baby Trap*, Heinrich Hanan, London.

Peel, J. and Potts, M. (1969), *Textbook of Contraceptive Practice*, Cambridge University Press.

Plowden Report (1967), *Children and their Primary Schools*, HMSO, London.

Pochin, J. (1969), *Without a Wedding Ring*, Constable, London.

Pohlman, E. H. (1965), '"Wanted" and "Unwanted": Toward less Ambiguous Definition', *Eugenics Quarterly*, vol. 12.

Pohlman, E. H. (1969), *Psychology of Birth Planning*, Schenkman, Cambridge, Mass.

Potts, M. (1973), *Responsible Abortions Services*, Pregnancy Advisory Services, London.

Rains, P. M. (1971), *Becoming an Unwed Mother*, Aldine Atherton, New York.

Rainwater, L. H. (1960), *And the Poor Get Children*, Quadrangle Paperbacks, Chicago.

Rapoport, R. and Rapoport, R. N. (1971), *Dual Career Families*, Pelican, Harmondsworth.

Raynor, L. (1971), *Giving up a Baby for Adoption*, Association of British Adoption Agencies, London.

Ripley, G. D. (1969), 'Health Education as a Basis for Medical Care. A Structured Course on Human Relationships', *Health Education Journal*, XXVIII, 3 Sept.

Rossi, A. (1973), *The Feminist Papers*, Columbia University Press, London.

Rossi, A. (1965), 'Equality between the Sexes: an Immodest Proposal' in R. J. Linton (ed.), *The Woman in America*, Houghton Mifflin, Boston.

Rowe, J. (1966), *Parents, Children and Adoption*, Routledge & Kegan Paul, London.

Rowe, J. (1975), 'A Children's Charter for Happiness?', *Community Care*, 5 Nov.

Rowe, J. and Lambert, L. (1973), *Children Who Wait*, Association of British Adoption Agencies, London.

Russell, J. K. (1970), 'Pregnancy in the Young Teenager', *The Practitioner*, March, vol. 204.

Rutter, M. (1972), *Maternal Deprivation Reassessed*, Penguin, Harmondsworth.

Schofield, M. (1968), *The Sexual Behaviour of Young People*, Penguin, Harmondsworth.

Schofield, M. (1973), *The Sexual Behaviour of Young Adults*, Allen Lane, The Penguin Press, London.

Seebohm Report (1968), *The Local Authority and Personal and Allied Social Services*, HMSO, London.

Select Committee on the Anti Discrimination Bill (1973), *Second Special Report*, HMSO, London.

Simms, M. (1970), 'Abortion Law Reform: How the Controversy Changed', *Criminal Law Review*, October.

Simms, M. (1973), *Report on Non-Medical Abortion Counselling*, Birth Control Trust, London.

Simms, M. (1974), 'Abortion Law and Medical Freedom', *British Journal of Criminology*, April.

Sinclair, L. (1956), *The Bridgeburn Days*, Gollancz, London

Smith, F. (1966), *Pregnancy in Adolescence: The Young Unmarried Father*, NCUMC, London.

Stevenson, O. (1972), *Claimant or Client?*, Allen & Unwin, London.

Streather, J. and Weir, S. (1974), *Social Insecurity*, CPAG.

Supplementary Benefits Handbook (1974), HMSO, London.

Timms, N. (1973), *At the Receiving End*, Routledge & Kegan Paul, London.

Titmuss, R. M. (1963), *Essays on The Welfare State*, Unwin University Books, London.

Tizard, B. (1974), *Preschool Education in Britain: a research review*, SSRC, London.

Todd Report (1968), Royal Commission of Medical Education, HMSO, London.

Tolstoy, L. N. (1973), *Anna Karenin*, Penguin, Harmondsworth.

Trasler, G. (1960), *In Place of Parents*, Routledge & Kegan Paul, London.

Triseliotis, J. (1971), 'Recent Developments Affecting Adopting Numbers and Adoption Practice', *British Journal of Social Work*, Autumn, vol. 1, no. 3.

Triseliotis, J. and Hall, E. (1971), 'Giving Consent to Adoption', *Social Work Today*, 2 December.

Truax, C. B. and Carkhuff, R. R. (1967), *Towards Effective Counselling and Psychotherapy*, Aldine, Chicago.

Venables, E. (1971), *Counselling*, National Marriage Guidance Council.

Vincent, C. (1961), *Unmarried Mothers*, Free Press, New York.

Waite, M. (1974), *Consultant Gynaecologists and Birth Control*, Birth Control Trust.

Wallis, J. H. (1973), *Personal Counselling*, Allen & Unwin, London.

Wallston, B. (1973), 'The Effects of Maternal Employment on Children', *Journal of Child Psychology and Psychiatry*, vol. 14, no. 2, June.

Warren, E. and Carstairs, V. (1974), 'Enquiry into the Role of Social Workers in the Care of Patients requesting Termination of Pregnancy', *Lane Report*, vol. 2, HMSO, London.

Weir, S. (1968), *A Study of Unmarried Mothers and their Children in Scotland*, Scottish Home and Health Department.

Williams, J. M. and Hindell, K. (1972), *Abortion and Contraception: A Study of Patients' Attitudes*, PEP Broadsheet 536, March.

Williams, R. (1969), *Working Wonders*, Hodder & Stoughton, London.

Wimperis, V. (1960), *The Unmarried Mother and Her Child*, Allen & Unwin, London.

Winnicott, D. W. (1963), 'The Value of Depression' in *Casework and Depression*, Association of Psychiatric Social Workers.

Woolf, M. (1971), *Family Intentions*, HMSO, London.

Wynn, M. (1964), *Fatherless Families*, Michael Joseph, London.

Yelloly, M. (1964), 'Social Casework with Unmarried Parents', unpublished thesis, University of Liverpool.

Yelloly, M. (1965), 'Factors Relating to the Adoption Decision by the Mothers of Illegitimate Infants', *Sociological Review*, vol. 13, no. 1, March.

Young, L. (1954), *Out of Wedlock*, McGraw-Hill, New York.

Young, M. (ed.) (1974), *Poverty Report*, Temple Smith, London.

Young, M. and Wilmott, P. (1957), *Family and Kinship in East London*, Routledge & Kegan Paul, London.

Yudkin, S. (1968), *0-5 A Report on the Case of Pre-school Children*, Allen & Unwin, London.

Yudkin, S. and Holme, A. (1969), *Working Mothers and their Children*, Sphere Books, London.

Index

Printed in the United States
by Baker & Taylor Publisher Services